DEMYSTIFYING WEIGHT LOSS

DEMYSTIFYING WEIGHT LOSS

A Concise Guide for Solving the Weight Loss Puzzle

Pamela Wartian Smith, M.D., MPH

Healthy Living Books, Inc.
TRAVERSE CITY, MICHIGAN

For information, please contact Healthy Living Books, Inc.,
575 S. Long Lake Road, Traverse City, MI 49684, (231) 943-4577.

First printing 2007

ISBN 978-0-9729767-5-6
LCCN 2007921996

To all of my patients
over the last thirty years
that I have served.
Thank you for
teaching me as much as
I have ever hoped
to teach you.

DISCLAIMER

This book is not intended to provide medical advice and is sold with the understanding that the publisher and the author are not liable for the misconception or misuse of information provided. The author and Healthy Living Books shall have neither liability nor responsibility to any person or entity with respect to any loss, damage, or injury caused or alleged to be caused directly or indirectly by the information contained in this book or the use of any products mentioned. Readers should not use any of the products discussed in this book without the advice of a medical professional. The information contained in this book is designed for information and education only and is not intended to prescribe treatment.

To see a board-certified practitioner in your area who is fellowship trained and specializes in anti-aging and functional medicine, contact:

- The Fellowship in Anti-Aging and Functional Medicine: 1-313-884-3229 or visit them on the web at: www.faafm.com
- The American Academy of Anti-Aging Physicians: 1-773-528-4333 or visit them on the web at: www.worldhealth.net
- The Institute for Functional Medicine: 1-253-858-4724 or visit them on the web at: www.fxmed.com
- The Center For Healthy Living: 1-888-884-3288 or visit us on the web at: www.cfhll.com

"The doctor of the future will give no medicine but will interest his patients in the care of the human frame, in diet, and in the cause and prevention of disease."

—Thomas A. Edison

CONTENTS

INTRODUCTION

The statistics focusing on obesity and being overweight are startling. An estimated 119 million American adults are overweight or obese (more than 20 pounds over ideal body weight).[1] It is projected that 73% of adults could be overweight or obese by 2008.[2] More than 9 million children or 15% of the younger population are either overweight or obese.[3] The rate of childhood obesity more than doubled from 1980 to the year 2000.[4]

Being overweight or obese increases your risk of 35 major diseases including diabetes, heart disease, stroke, arthritis, sleep apnea, and cancer.[5] In a recent article in the *Journal of the American Medical Association*, smoking was the leading cause of mortality. However, the article points out that poor diet and physical inactivity may soon overtake tobacco as the leading cause of death.[6]

There is indeed an epidemic of weight gain and obesity in the United States. According to the Centers for Disease Control and the National Institutes of Health, obesity was the attributable cause of approximately 112,000 deaths annually in a study published in April 2005.[7] The conclusion of this study was that members of this generation, those now age 35 and younger, might be the first in history to die younger than their parents.

The direct and indirect costs of obesity, including medical services and lost productivity, amount to more than $117 billion dollars a year according to the U.S. Department of Health and Human Services.[8] A study published in 2002 showed that obesity increases the cost of healthcare for inpatient services by 36% and medication costs increase by 77% compared to people of ideal weight.[9]

The average American adult gains 3 pounds a year. It does not sound like much, but imagine yourself ten years from now. This book focuses on the multifactorial reasons that people gain weight and have a hard time losing it. It is not just simply what you put into your mouth. Yes, calories in should equal calories out; however, there are reasons why some people crave certain foods and why some people burn calories faster than others. This book explores these reasons.

Have your healthcare practitioner or exercise physiologist do a body fat analysis on you, which is an indication of your lean body mass. This will aid both of you in developing a customized program to help you to achieve your goal of weight loss.

Ideal Body Fat Percentage for Women and Men

Women 19–23%
Men 14–18%

Foods you eat communicate with your cells, and the message sent can be either beneficial or detrimental to your long-term health. This includes weight loss. Let us look at how this communication occurs.

Allergies and Weight Loss

1

Weight gain may be due to allergies to food or food intolerances. Sixty percent of the U.S. suffers from undetected food allergies.[1] If you are eating foods to which you are allergic, immune complexes form in your body. To minimize this reaction, the body retains fluid to try to dilute the immune complexes and make them less concentrated. This excess fluid contributes to weight gain.

Many people crave foods they are allergic to. A great book on inflammation that also has a wonderful chapter on allergies is *Stopping Inflammation, Relieving the Cause of Degenerative Diseases*, by Nancy Appleton.[2] Physical symptoms of food allergies are listed below:[3, 4]

- Abdominal pain
- Aching muscles
- Acne
- Addictions
- Anemia
- Arthritis
- Asthma
- Athlete's foot
- Bad breath
- Bed-wetting
- Blackouts
- Bloating
- Blood sugar problems
- Bloody stools
- Blurred vision
- Breast pain
- Bursitis
- Canker sores
- Celiac disease
- Chronic bladder infections
- Chronic fatigue syndrome
- Chronic or recurrent infections
- Coated tongue
- Colitis
- Compulsive drinking

- Constant hunger
- Constipation
- Coughing
- Cravings for certain foods
- Difficulty in swallowing
- Dizziness
- Eczema
- Excessive thirst
- Excessive or no sweating
- Failure of newborn infants to develop
- Fainting
- Fatigue
- Feeling drained
- Flushes
- Frequent need to urinate
- Gall bladder disease
- Gas
- Gastritis
- Gritty feeling in eyes
- Headaches, all types
- Heavy body odor
- High/low blood pressure
- Hives
- Hyperactivity
- Indigestion, recurring
- Infant colic
- Inflammation
- Insomnia
- Intestinal bleeding
- Irritability
- Irritable bowel syndrome
- Itching
- Itchy or red eyes and/or ears
- Lethargy
- Loss of appetite
- Lower back pain
- Malabsorption of food
- Menstrual problems
- Metallic taste
- Mouth ulcers
- Multiple sclerosis
- Muscle aches and cramps
- Muscle tremors
- Nausea
- Palpitations (heart racing)
- Persistent cough
- Poor balance
- Postnasal drip
- Premenstrual problems
- Racing pulse
- Rashes
- Recurrent bronchitis
- Recurrent croup
- Recurrent ear infections
- Restless leg syndrome
- Rhinitis
- Schizophrenia
- Seizures
- Sensitivity to light and noise
- Sinusitis
- Sleep disturbances
- Sore, itching, puffy or burning eyes
- Sore tongue
- Stiff neck
- Styes
- Systemic lupus erythematosus (SLE)

- Temperature fluctuations
- Thrush
- Tics
- Ulcerative colitis
- Ulcers
- Vertigo
- Vomiting
- Watering eyes
- Weight gain or loss
- Wheezing

You may not realize you have a food allergy. When you intake a food you are allergic to, it sets off a response in the body. This response releases numerous chemical reactions including neurotransmitter responses. You initially get a "high" from eating foods that start an allergic-inflammatory response in your body. You get addicted to this "high" feeling. You may not develop other symptoms until hours or even days later. Consequently, you do not relate the ingestion of this food to a substance that you are allergic to. An IgE blood test (the typically studied immunoglobulin) is not the best way to evaluate whether you have a food allergy. Many people have a food hypersensitivity, which is mediated through another immunoglobulin pathway called IgG. A complete blood screen is available from laboratories that specialize in this kind of testing (see Appendix). If you think this may be a problem for you, see a fellowship trained anti-aging and functional medicine practitioner who can order this test. (For availability, see the beginning of this book.) They can test your blood to see what foods you are allergic to or place you on an allergy elimination diet, which will determine which foods you are sensitive to. Avoiding these foods will help with weight loss.

The top four foods that cause allergies are wheat, dairy products, soy, and eggs. Other common foods that frequently result in allergic responses are barley, beef, chocolate, citrus, coffee, nuts (including peanuts), rye, seafood, sugar, tea, and tomatoes.[5]

The brain is also affected by the mast cell production that occurs when you have an allergic reaction. Therefore, your thoughts and actions may also be governed by this allergic-inflammatory response. Symptoms of allergic reactions involving the brain are listed below:[6]

- Aggression
- Anger for no apparent reason
- Anxiety
- Attention deficit disorder (ADD) with or without hyperactivity
- Changes in handwriting
- Chewing clothes and bedclothes
- Clumsiness
- Compulsive behavior
- Confusion, disorientation, "brain fog," and blankness
- Daydreaming
- Delusions
- Depression
- Detached or unreal feeling
- Difficulty waking up
- Dyslexia and other learning disabilities
- Emotional sensitivity
- Erratic behavior
- Fearfulness
- Hallucinations
- Hearing without comprehension
- Hyperactivity, including fidgeting
- Impatience
- Inability to be pleased
- Indecisiveness
- Indifference to work, clothes, hygiene, friends, etc.
- Irresponsibility
- Irritability
- Lethargy (mental and physical)
- Loss of sex drive
- Math, spelling, and reading errors
- Memory loss
- Mood swings
- Morbid mood
- Nightmares
- Not open to reason
- Panic attacks
- Paranoia
- Phobias
- Poor self-image
- Poor work habits
- Restlessness
- Screaming attacks
- Slow metabolism
- Slurred, stammering, and/or stuttering speech
- Suicidal inclinations
- Sulkiness
- Tenseness
- Uncooperativeness
- Weepiness

Research has shown that food allergies affect the limbic region of the brain. This area is associated with the hunger response, consequently affecting your ability to lose weight.[7] Furthermore, food allergy responses act as false kinins, which cause inflammation and interfere with neurotransmitter function (see Chapters 9 and 15, on inflammation and neurotransmitters). These are other mechanisms whereby food allergies can affect weight gain. Allergic reactions also directly affect the central nervous system and mood.[8] There have been many books, much research, and numerous articles on the psychological component of obesity. It will be looked at throughout this book under several categories.

Stress Hormones and Weight Loss

2

Stress is another factor that can lead to weight gain. The most stressful jobs are the following:[1]

- Construction worker
- Secretary
- Laboratory technician
- Waiter or waitress
- Machine operator
- Farmer
- House painter
- Mid-level manager
- Foreman/supervisor

What do all of these jobs have in common? The answer is lack of control. Some stress is good in your life. It lets you know you are alive. But too much stress can be detrimental to the body. Excess stress can cause depletion of minerals and other nutrients. B vitamins, vitamins C and E, calcium, magnesium, phosphorus, and potassium may become depleted.

The body may develop symptoms of stress, which can be divided into four categories: physical, behavioral, emotional, and cognitive. Dr. Herbert Benson in his book *The Relaxation Response* discusses these symptoms.[2]

Physical symptoms:

- Headaches
- Indigestion
- Stomachaches
- Sweaty palms
- Sleep difficulties
- Dizziness
- Tight neck, shoulders
- Racing heart
- Restlessness
- Tiredness
- Ringing in ears
- Back pain

Behavioral symptoms

- Excess smoking
- Bossiness
- Grinding of teeth at night
- Overuse of alcohol
- Compulsive gum chewing
- Attitude critical of others
- Compulsive eating
- Inability to get things done

Emotional symptoms

- Crying
- Nervousness, anxiety
- Boredom—no meaning to anything
- Edginess—ready to explode
- Feeling powerless to change things
- Overwhelming sense of pressure
- Anger
- Loneliness
- Unhappiness for no reason
- Easily upset

Cognitive symptoms

- Trouble thinking clearly
- Forgetfulness
- Lack of creativity
- Memory loss
- Inability to make decisions
- Thoughts of running away
- Constant worry
- Loss of sense of humor

If you feel competence, power, and control during the stress, this alters your perception and actions. Stress may actually increase your ability to focus and concentrate. This is called "being in the zone." Here, you feel competent and powerful because you are in control even though you may be under extreme stress. This is what world-class athletes feel when they are winning and emergency room physicians experience when they are able to remember all of the cases going on in the emergency room at the same time without having to review the charts again. How you respond to stress is the key. You may not be able to change the stressor, but you can change how you respond to it.

Many people eat more food when they are stressed. When you are stressed, your hormonal response in the body changes. The two hormones that govern stress are DHEA and cortisol.

DHEA is a hormone made by your adrenal glands. A small amount is also made in your brain and skin. DHEA production declines with age, starting in your late twenties. By the age of 70 you make one-fourth of the amount you made earlier. DHEA makes your other sex hormones.

Functions of DHEA in your body:[3]

- Promotes weight loss
- Decreases cholesterol
- Decreases formation of fatty deposits
- Prevents blood clots
- Increases bone growth
- Increases brain function
- Increases sense of well-being
- Helps you deal with stress
- Supports your immune system
- Helps your body repair itself and maintain tissues
- Decreases allergic reactions

Low DHEA can be due to:[4]

- Stress
- Menopause
- Andropause (male menopause)
- Aging
- Smoking (Nicotine inhibits the production of an enzyme, 11-beta-hydroxylase, which is needed to make DHEA).[5,6]

Replacement of DHEA can:[7]

- Increase muscle strength and lean body mass
- Activate immune function
- Increase quality of life
- Improve sleep
- Increase feeling of wellness
- Decrease joint soreness
- Increase sensitivity of insulin
- Decrease triglycerides
- Stop the damaging effects of stress

DHEA has been shown to have a protective effect against cancer, diabetes, obesity, increased cholesterol, heart disease, and autoimmune diseases.[8,9,10]

You can overdose on DHEA. Women are more sensitive to the effects of DHEA and need less DHEA than men.

The following symptoms of too much DHEA include:

- Fatigue
- Anger
- Depression
- Deepening of voice
- Insomnia
- Mood changes
- Weight gain
- Facial hair
- Acne
- Sugar cravings
- Restless sleep
- Irritability

When the body is first stressed, DHEA elevates, and it is supposed to go right back down to normal levels. If you stay stressed, then after a while, instead of having excess DHEA, you make too little. This phenomenon occurs because your body is no longer able to make enough DHEA to keep up with the level of stress that you are experiencing.

Cortisol is the only hormone in your body that increases with age. Cortisol, like DHEA, is made by your adrenal glands.

Cortisol is involved in the following ways in the body:[11,12]

- Balancing blood sugar
- Weight control
- Immune system response
- Bone turnover rate
- Stress reaction
- Sleep
- Protein synthesis
- Mood and thoughts
- Influences testosterone/estrogen ratio
- Affects pituitary/thyroid/adrenal system

Stress increases cortisol as do depression and high progestin intake (birth control pills and synthetic progesterone).[13]

The following are long-term consequences of elevated cortisol:[14,15]

- Weight gain
- Binge eating
- Decreased immune system
- Increased osteoporosis risk
- Fatigue
- Irritability
- Sugar cravings
- Shakiness between meals
- Confusion
- Sleep disturbances
- Low energy
- Night sweats and hot flashes
- Increased blood pressure
- Increased cholesterol
- Elevated triglycerides
- High blood sugar
- Increased insulin/insulin resistance
- Increased infections
- Thin skin
- Easy bruising
- Muscle weakness

Abnormal cortisol levels are associated with the following conditions:[16]

- Weight gain/obesity
- Chronic fatigue syndrome
- Fibromyalgia
- Depression
- Impotence
- Anorexia nervosa
- Panic disorders
- PMS
- Infertility
- Sleep disorders
- Osteoporosis
- Heart disease
- Menopause/andropause (male menopause)

All of the hormones in your body are designed to work in balance together. In order for you to enjoy good health and lose weight, they all have to be balanced and at an optimal level. In other words, your hormones are a symphony, and they have to play in tune for you to be healthy and be at an ideal weight. If your cortisol is increased, it decreases the making of progesterone and its activity.[17] Cortisol competes with progesterone for common receptors in women. Furthermore, when cortisol is high, it makes your thyroid hormone become more bound and therefore less active in both men and women, which can add to weight gain.[18]

When your adrenal glands are in a state of "emergency," you do not feel well. You may reach for coffee, soft drinks, or sugar for a source of energy. This makes the situation worse. If your adrenal glands stay stimulated, you cause them to weaken or "burn out." Then, your cortisol and DHEA levels drop. This syndrome of low cortisol and DHEA is called adrenal fatigue. It is a sub-optimal functioning of the adrenal glands due to their inability to keep pace with the demands placed upon them by the total amount of stress. This is not Addison's Disease, in which your body is totally depleted of cortisol. With adrenal fatigue, the body makes enough cortisol to stay alive but not enough for your body to function optimally. Adrenal fatigue is seldom detected by most health professionals. You need to see a practitioner that specializes in anti-aging and functional medicine. A must-read is the book *Adrenal Fatigue* by Dr. James Wilson.[19] Adrenal fatigue is very common.[20] There are many clinical symptoms and conditions associated with adrenal fatigue.[21] They include:

- Weight gain
- Decreased immunity
- Lack of stamina
- Emotional paralysis
- PTSD (post-traumatic stress disorder)
- Poor wound healing
- Increased susceptibility to infection
- Weak cardiac function
- Alcoholism and drug addiction
- Hypoglycemia
- Unresponsive hypothyroidism
- Persistence of low thyroid symptoms despite treatment

- Slow recovery from illness, injury, trauma, stressful situations
- Collapse after hearing bad news
- Loss of motivation or initiative
- General feeling of "unwellness"
- Persistent feeling of being overwhelmed
- Progressively poorer athletic performance
- Craves salt and foods high in salt
- Often craves food high in fat
- Feels better with high fat diet
- Often uses high fat or sugary foods with caffeine to drive themselves
- Often becomes hypoglycemic (low blood sugar), especially under stress
- Intolerance to high potassium foods, especially in the morning
- Often does not handle carbohydrates well without fats or protein
- Needs to lie down or rest after sessions of psychological or emotional stress
- Decreased sex drive
- Syncope or lightheadedness when rising rapidly from a sitting or lying position
- Chronic fatigue
- Increased apathy or interest in things
- Hyperventilation, frequent sighing, gasping-type of breath
- Develops allergies or sensitivities
- Chemical intolerances
- Tendency toward chronic allergic states (skin conditions, rash, dermatitis, etc.)
- Nervousness or irritability
- Inability to concentrate—especially before lunch
- Excessive fears and apprehensions

- Easily confused
- Muscular weakness—lack of stamina, tires too easily
- Mild constipation or diarrhea that increases under stress
- Alternating constipation and diarrhea
- Bowel movements may tend to be dry and hard
- Dull tummy ache for no apparent reason
- Chronic colds, coughs, hay fever
- Frequent recurring respiratory infections
- Increased PMS, peri-menopausal, menopausal, or andropausal symptoms
- Increased incidence and severity of some asthmas
- Slow recovery from trauma or illness
- Less social and more symptoms after trauma or illness

If you have adrenal fatigue, you may have experienced it after a long period of stress or one severe stressful event such as a divorce or car accident. Frequently, you have driven yourself to exhaustion and have been overworked with no play time or relaxation. Caregivers frequently experience adrenal fatigue. Over-exercise or intense participation in competitive sports may also be a common history. Patients frequently tell me that "they were never the same after _______ happened to them." Decreased sexual drive, missed promotions and opportunities at work, martial discord, and lost productivity at work and home are also common scenarios that patients describe who have adrenal fatigue. Extreme fatigue is also very common. The more stressors and the longer they last, the larger the cumulative stress load.

Dr. Wilson describes a daily energy pattern that is common with people with adrenal fatigue.[22] You may have morning fatigue, with difficulty waking early in the A.M., and not feel really awake until after 10:00 A.M. Usually, you feel much better and more awake after the noon meal and again have a low time in the afternoon between 2:00 and 4:00 P.M. You may feel your best after 6:00 P.M.

At night, you may be tired again around 9:00–10:00 but resist going to bed. You get a second burst of energy commonly at 11:00 P.M., and it may last until 1:00–2:00 in the morning. Your most refreshing sleep is usually between 7:00 and 9:00 A.M. You do your best work late at night and have a hard time getting up the next morning.

Many physicians and other healthcare providers have adrenal fatigue. Aggravating factors include constant stress at home and/or work stress, poor dietary habits, unhappy relationships at work or home, lack of exercise, insufficient enjoyable activities, no control over how you spend your time, and excess responsibility.[23]

Lab testing for adrenal fatigue can be done by blood, urine, or saliva. Usually, blood reference ranges are too broad and therefore do not adequately measure adrenal fatigue. A 24-hour urine test may also be done, but it does not give you the times of day that the adrenal fatigue may be at its worst. Consequently, saliva testing is considered to be the preferred method of measuring cortisol levels.

For women, decreased estradiol (estrogen) is, in itself, a stressor to the body. It causes an increase in cortisol because estradiol causes a decrease in optimal function of norepinephrine, serotonin, dopamine, and acetylcholine, which are neurotransmitters responsible for communication between the cells (see Chapter 15 on neurotransmitters).[24]

Consequently, there is a link between stress and obesity. Stress leads to increased cortisol concentrations, which induce increased food intake. Stress may contribute to abdominal obesity characterized by increases in cortisol and leptin concentrations.[25] Growth hormone and its effects on cortisol metabolism may be related to the pathogenesis of central obesity as well.[26] Cortisol also stimulates enzymes in fat cells, which increases abdominal fat storage.[27]

Men have the same responses to stress as women with the same changes in hormonal function and depletion of minerals and nutrients. Depletion of testosterone for a male can cause him to have a long-term stress response.

As you can see from the above, stress and the body's response to stress can cause weight gain and obesity. Cortisol promotes the release of neuropeptide Y, which is a brain chemical that stimulates the body to increase intake of carbohydrates. Therefore, in order to lose weight and keep it off, it is important to have normal DHEA and cortisol levels.

When you are stressed or you know you are about to enter a stressful time in your life, it is important to eat well. Limiting caffeine and sugar intake is very helpful. The following are foods that have been found to help with stress:[28]

- Almonds
- Apples
- Bananas
- Cabbage
- Cantaloupe
- Carrots
- Chicken (skinless white meat, broiled)
- Figs
- Grapefruit
- Grapes
- Mushrooms
- Onions
- Oranges
- Pears
- Pineapple
- Plums
- Potatoes
- Raisins
- Salmon
- String beans
- Tomatoes
- Turkey

The right diet can also repair the damage that stress has on the body. Good food helps the cells in the body communicate well with each other. Fad and crash diets cause stress to your body. Eating programs that include too little calories also cause stress to the body and may promote weight loss initially, but as soon as you go back to eating a regular number of calories, you gain weight.

Many people suffer from adrenal fatigue. A lifestyle change is paramount to treat this condition. Overbooking is a frequent issue. Stress reduction techniques are key in helping to heal your body. Prayer, meditation, tai chi, yoga, chi gong, exercise, and massage have all been found to aid in the healing of the adrenal glands. Music is also good therapy. Healing herbs, nutrients, and adrenal extracts are also part of the treatment used for adrenal fatigue. Listed below are adrenal support supplements that have been found to work.[29,30,31,32,33,34,35,36,37] See the Appendix for pharmaceutical grade neutraceutical companies that will help your healthcare practitioner treat abnormal DHEA and cortisol levels.

Adrenal support supplements:

• Glycyrrhiza	600 mg twice a day
• Ashwaghanda	160 mg twice a day
• Rheumania root	2,000 mg twice a day
• Ginseng	200 mg twice a day
• Cordyceps	400 mg twice a day
• Rhodiola	50 mg twice a day
• B vitamins	100 mg twice a day
• Vitamin C	1,000–2,000 mg
• L-carnitine	1,000–3,000 mg
• Magnesium	400–600 mg
• Phosphatidylserine	300 mg
• Holy Basil	
• Bacopa	
• Amino acids	as per lab results

Likewise, short-term use of cortef, a medication, is also helpful to optimize DHEA and cortisol levels.

In order to be healthy, you have to be physically healthy, psychologically healthy, and spiritually healthy. Whatever religion you may be, do not carry burdens that God is supposed to carry for you. Spiritual health is important in helping the body have a healthy response to stress.

Female Hormones and Weight Loss

3

Female hormonal disorders, such as PMS (premenstrual syndrome) and PCOS (polycystic ovarian syndrome), are also associated with weight gain. Likewise, the average weight gain at peri-menopause and menopause is 20 pounds.

PMS

PMS is a hormonal disorder that is characterized by the monthly recurrence of physical or psychological symptoms during the two weeks prior to the menstrual cycle and the subsiding of those symptoms when the cycle begins.

Some symptoms of PMS affect weight gain. These include: abdominal bloating, appetite changes, and salt and sugar cravings. There are numerous other symptoms of PMS as well.

PMS can be treated with a better than 90% success rate. There are no definitive diagnostic tests that confirm a diagnosis of PMS, but a low progesterone level on days 12–14 of the menstrual cycle, confirmed by saliva testing, very commonly is associated with this syndrome. There is no clear course of development. However, something in the person's life interferes with the pituitary-ovarian feedback loop, and it decreases the supply of progesterone. Precipitating factors for PMS include: oral contraceptives due to the progestin (synthetic progesterone), pregnancies, miscarriages and abortions, and tubal ligations. Studies have shown that after tubal ligation women have higher estrogen and lower progesterone levels in the second half of their cycle.[1] Likewise, partial hysterectomy may be a precipitating factor for PMS due to the decreased supply of blood to the ovaries post hysterectomy. Low blood-sugar levels and caffeine also are key factors in PMS.

There are several treatment modalities that have proven to be successful for PMS, such as limiting a high-salt diet, magnesium, vitamin A, increasing exercise, and herbal therapies like black cohosh and chasteberry.[2] Since PMS is a state that is affected by low progesterone levels, progesterone supplementation has been found to be helpful. This should be with bio-identical progesterone, which is the same chemical structure that the body makes. This is also called natural progesterone and is a prescription made by a compounding pharmacy to be used days 12–24 of the menstrual cycle. If the person has insomnia, then progesterone is best taken as a pill so that it affects the GABA receptors in the brain. It will then have a calming effect and allow a person to sleep better. Otherwise, transdermally (on the skin) applied progesterone is very effective for the treatment of PMS. There is also a subset of women who have low estradiol and normal progesterone levels associated with PMS. For these women, progesterone will not work. Low levels of estradiol are associated with neurotransmitter changes including dopamine, norepinephrine, and epinephrine depletion. Furthermore, a rapid rise and fall in estrogen levels can affect serotonin production (see Chapter 15 on neurotransmitters). This may trigger depression and changes in eating pattern. For this subset of women, herbal therapies can be more effective.

PCOS

PCOS stands for polycystic ovarian disease, which is characterized by irregular cycles or absence of menstruation and excess testosterone (androgen) production. Signs and symptoms of PCOS include:[3]

- Obesity
- Irregular or absent menstrual cycles
- Infertility/recurrent miscarriage
- Hirsutism (excessive body hair)
- Oily skin/acne
- Alopecia (hair loss)
- Skin tags
- Depression

Other symptoms of PCOS include cysts on the ovaries, high testosterone levels, elevated insulin level or insulin resistance, elevated LH (luteinizing hormone), decreased sex hormone binding globulin, abnormal lipid profile (cholesterol, triglycerides), and hypertension (high blood pressure).

Many scientists believe that PCOS has a hereditary component.[4,5] There is also some suggestion in the medical literature that women with PCOS are born with a gene that triggers elevated levels of testosterone or insulin.[6,7] Furthermore, studies have shown that the high levels of testosterone and insulin in patients with PCOS are linked. This link is a gene called follistatin. In the body, follistatin has two functions. It plays a role in the development of the ovaries and it is also needed to make insulin.[8] Stress can also be a contributing factor to PCOS.[9] Recent studies have shown that many women with PCOS cannot process cortisol effectively. This may lead to elevated cortisol levels.[10] Likewise, women who are under a lot of stress make too much prolactin. This may affect the ability of the ovaries to produce hormones in a balanced manner.[11]

Polycystic ovarian syndrome is a risk factor for other major diseases, including obesity and insulin resistance, which can lead to diabetes.[12,13,14,15,16] Studies have shown that women with PCOS store fat better and burn calories at a slower rate than women who do not have PCOS.[17,18,19]

The treatment of PCOS includes medications, fiber, eating foods from a low glycemic index program, reducing stress, and increasing the intake of essential fatty acids, like fish oil, and antioxidants. Drugs that are menstrual regulators can also be helpful, such as oral contraceptives and natural progesterone. I have found bio-identical (natural progesterone) to be very helpful. Herbal remedies like fenugreek, gymnema sylvestre, cinnamon, black cohosh, and chasteberries have been useful to treat PCOS. Nutrients that help lower blood sugar and treat insulin resistance should also be employed. They include:[20]

• Chromium picolinate	400–600 micrograms
• Alpha lipoic acid	200–600 mg
• CLA	1,000–3,000 mg
• Zinc	25–50 mg
• Taurine	1,000–3,000 mg
• Magnesium	400–800 mg
• Biotin	4–8 mg
• Vanadium	20–50 mg
• Vitamin D	400–2,000 IU
• Coenzyme Q10	30–300 mg
• B complex	50–100 mg
• Vitamin C	1,000–3,000 mg
• Manganese	5–10 mg
• Inositol	

- Lentils, chickpeas, and broccoli all decrease insulin levels.

High doses of niacin should be avoided in people with PCOS since it can worsen insulin sensitivity. A great book to read is *The PCOS Protection Plan* by Colette Harris and Theresa Cheung.[21]

Peri-menopause and Menopause

For more mature women, hormones likewise play a role in weight gain. As women go through peri-menopause and menopause, many women put on extra pounds. In order to lose weight and keep it off, a woman's sex hormones have to be balanced and replaced if lost. One size does not fit all. What each woman needs is as unique to her as her fingerprints. Therefore, her treatment should be customized to her own individual needs. The results of the Women's Health Initiative Study highlights the problems associated with "one-size-fits-all" medicine. If the body is deficient in hormones, they should be replaced with bio-identical hormones. For a longer discussion on the subject, see my book, *HRT: The Answers*.[22]

Estrogen has 400 functions in the body. One of those is to make insulin work better, which helps to keep a woman's blood sugar normal.[23,24,25,26] This aids in weight loss. Estrogen also helps the formation of neurotransmitters in the brain, such as serotonin, which decreases depression, irritability, and anxiety. Abnormal levels of serotonin and other neurotransmitters can lead women to eat "comfort foods" that can also cause weight gain.[27,28] The body has receptor sites for estrogen everywhere, including the brain, muscles, bone, bladder, gut, uterus, ovaries, vagina, breast, eyes, heart, lungs, and blood vessels.

The following are symptoms of low estrogen levels:

- Thinner skin
- More wrinkles/aging skin
- Decrease in breast size
- Stress incontinence
- Oily skin
- Acne
- Decreased sex drive
- Decreased dexterity
- Increase insulin resistance
- Vaginal dryness
- Decreased memory
- Osteoporosis or osteopenia
- Urinary tract infections
- Elevated cholesterol

One can have too much estrogen in the body. Estrogen levels must be in balance with other hormones, such as progesterone. Dr. John Lee coined the phrase "estrogen dominance" to describe symptoms of estrogen excess.[29] One of the main symptoms of too much estrogen is weight gain, especially around the abdomen, hips, and thighs.

Other symptoms of estrogen excess (some of which can also add to difficulties in weight control) include:[30,31]

- Cervical dysplasia
- Decreased sexual interest
- Depression with anxiety or agitation
- Increased risk of cancer of the uterus
- Water retention
- Headaches
- Poor sleep
- Panic attacks
- Swollen breasts
- Heavy periods
- Increased risk of breast cancer
- Increased risk of auto-immune diseases
- Hypothyroidism (increases the binding of thyroid hormone)
- Fatigue
- Fibrocystic breasts
- Irritability
- Mood swings
- Uterine fibroids
- Bloating

Estrogen dominance can result from the overproduction of estrogen or from an imbalance of progesterone to estrogen. The symptoms of estrogen excess may also be the result of the transformation of estrogens by the liver, rather than with the absolute amount of estrogen in the system. (See section on estrogen metabolism.)

Causes of estrogen dominance:[32]

- Taking too much estrogen
- Impaired elimination of estrogen
- Lack of exercise
- Diet low in grains and fiber
- Environmental estrogens
- Elevation of 16-hydroxyestrone

The kinds of estrogen a woman makes are also important. Women make three main Estrogens:

- E1 called estrone
- E2 called estradiol
- E3 called estriol

Estrone (E1)

Estrone is the main estrogen the body makes postmenopausally. High levels stimulate breast and uterine tissue, and many researchers believe it may be related to an increased risk of breast and uterine cancer.[33,34]

Before menopause, estrone is made by the ovaries, adrenal glands, liver, and fat cells. Estrone, pre-menopausally, is converted to estradiol in the ovaries. Postmenopausally, little estrone becomes estradiol since the ovaries greatly decrease function. Estrone, in later years, is then made in the fat cells and to a lesser degree in the liver and adrenal glands.[35] Therefore, the more body fat a woman has, the more estrone she makes. Consequently, obese women have an increased estrone to estradiol ratio, which predisposes them to breast cancer.[36] Also, routine alcohol consumption decreases ovarian hormone levels and shifts the estrogen to estrone.[37,38]

Estradiol (E2)

Estradiol is the strongest estrogen. It is 12 times stronger than estrone and 80 times stronger than estriol. It is the main estrogen women make before menopause. Most of estradiol is made in the ovaries. High levels of E2 are associated with an increased risk of breast and uterine cancer. Estradiol is the estrogen women lose at menopause. However, two-thirds of postmenopausal women up to the age of 80 continue to make some estradiol.[39] Estradiol levels are lower in women who have had a surgical procedure affecting their ovaries. In other words, even if a woman has a tubal ligation or a partial hysterectomy (ovaries are left in), she may still have a decrease in her hormonal function and have symptoms of hormonal loss.[40] Estradiol is responsible for most of the 400 functions that estrogen has in the body.

Estriol E3

Estriol has a much less stimulating effect on the breast and uterine lining than estrone or estradiol. Estriol has been shown not to promote breast cancer, and considerable evidence exists to show that it protects against it.[41,42,43,44] Asian and vegetarian women have high levels of estriol and much lower rates of breast cancer.[45] Estriol (E3) does not have the bone, heart, or brain protection, however, that estradiol does.[46,47] Therefore, most women need to have both E2 and E3 estrogens replaced. Any percentage can be used of these two estrogens since the dosage is individualized per patient. It is made by a compounding pharmacy that specializes in making medications that are customized per person. For availability of a compounding pharmacist, see the Appendix.

It is necessary that a woman have her levels of all three estrogens measured before she begins hormone replacement and regularly thereafter, to help maintain the correct level of replacement.

How a person takes estrogen is also important. I recommend giving estrogen only by the transdermal route. This is through the skin. Estrogen taken orally can increase carbohydrate cravings and increase weight gain.[48]

Estrogen given by mouth can also:[49,50]

- Increase blood pressure
- Elevate triglycerides
- Increase estrone (E1)
- Cause gallstones
- Elevate liver enzymes
- Decrease growth hormone (the hormone that keeps you younger)
- Interrupt tryptophan metabolism and consequently serotonin metabolism (Serotonin helps keep one calm and happy.)
- Elevate sex hormone binding globulin (can decrease testosterone)

There is a growing body of research showing that it is not simply the amount of total estrogen circulating in the body that is critical to one's health. How estrogen is broken down or metabolized in the body may also play an important role in the cause of a variety of estrogen-dependent conditions, including osteoporosis, autoimmune disorders, and cancer.

After menopause, the metabolism of estrogen can change. Consequently, a person may respond differently to estrogen.[51] Estrogen is metabolized in the body by the liver in the following ways:

Two major competing pathways:

2-hydroxyestrone
16-hydroxyestrone

One minor pathway:

4-hydroxyestrone

2-hydroxyestrone is sometimes called the "good" estrogen.[52] It does not stimulate the cells to divide which can damage the DNA and cause tumor growth.[53] Furthermore, by latching onto available estrogen cell receptors, 2-hydroxyestrone may exhibit a blocking action that prevents stronger estrogen products from gaining a foothold into the cells. Therefore, 2-hydroxyestrone is suggested to be anti-cancerous.[54]

The other major pathway whereby estrogen is metabolized is 16-hydroxyestrone. This metabolite is much more active and powerful. It has a strong stimulatory effect. 16-hydroxyestrone binds to special receptors inside the cells that can increase the rate of DNA synthesis. 16-hydroxyestone is proposed to have significant estrogenic activity and to be associated with an increased risk of breast cancer.[55,56,57,58,59,60,61,62,63,64,65] A woman's body does need a small amount of 16-hydroxyestrone to maintain bone structure. Therefore, the ratio between 2- and 16-hydroxyestrone is also important.

A minor pathway of estrogen metabolism is 4-hydroxyestrone. It may also enhance cancer development. 4-hydroxyestrone may directly damage DNA by causing breaks in the molecular strands of DNA.[66] Consequently, it is important to have the metabolization of estrogen measured. See Appendix for availability of labs that provide this testing.

Progesterone is also one of the sex hormones that a woman makes that declines with peri-menopause and menopause. Low levels of progesterone are also seen with PMS, PCOS, and postpartum depression. It is made in the ovaries before menopause. After menopause, some progesterone is made in the adrenal glands.

The following are symptoms of decreased progesterone:

- Anxiety
- Depression
- Irritability
- Mood swings
- Insomnia
- Pain and inflammation
- Osteoporosis
- Decreased HDL (good cholesterol)
- Excessive menstruation

There are many causes of low progesterone, including:

- Impaired production secondary to hormonal changes
- Low luteinizing hormone (LH)
- Increased prolactin production
- Stress[67]
- Antidepressants[68]
- Excessive arginine consumption[69]
- Sugar[70]
- Saturated fat[71]
- Deficiency of vitamins A, B6, and C and zinc[72,73]
- Decreased thyroid hormone

Synthetic progesterone is called progestin. It is very different from natural progesterone since it does not have the same chemical structure as the progesterone that the body makes on its own. Natural progesterone is biologically identical to what the body produces. Consequently, progestins do not reproduce the actions of natural progesterone.[74]

Let's first look at progestins (synthetic progesterone). Progestins are contained in birth control pills, Provera, Prempro, and other synthetic hormone replacement.

The following are side effects of progestins (synthetic progesterone) that do not occur with natural (bio-identical) progesterone.[75,76,77] Some of these affect weight.

- Increased appetite[78]
- Weight gain[79]
- Fluid retention
- Irritability
- Depression
- Headache
- Decreased energy
- Bloating
- Breast tenderness
- Decreased sexual interest
- Rash

- Acne
- Hair loss
- Nausea
- Insomnia
- Breakthrough bleeding/spotting
- Interferes with the body's own production of progesterone
- Does not help balance estrogen
- Remains in the body longer
- Can cause spasm of the coronary (heart) arteries[80]
- Stops the protective effects estrogen has on the heart[81,82,83,84,85]
- Attaches to many of the body's receptor sites, not just the progesterone receptors (long-term effects are unknown)[86]
- Cannot help make estrogen and testosterone
- May make the symptoms of progesterone loss worse
- Increased LDL (bad cholesterol)
- Decreased HDL (good cholesterol)
- Protects only the uterus from cancer[87,88]
- Counteracts many of the positive effects of estrogen on serotonin[89]

A recent study has shown that the use of synthetic progesterone increases the risk of breast cancer by 800% as compared to the use of estrogen alone.[90,91,92,93]

Progesterone's (natural) effect not seen with progestins:[94]

- Helps the body use and eliminate fats
- Helps balance estrogen
- Leaves the body quickly
- Helps sleep
- Has a natural calming effect[95]
- Lowers high blood pressure
- Lowers cholesterol
- May protect against breast cancer
- Increases scalp hair
- Normalizes libido

- Helps balance fluids in the cells
- Increases the beneficial effects of estrogens on blood vessel dilation in atherosclerotic plaques (hardening of the arteries)[96,97,98]
- Has an anti-proliferative effect (decreases the rate of cancer) on the progesterone receptors not just the ones in the uterus[99,100]
- Does not change the good effect estrogen has on blood flow[101]
- Increases metabolic rate[102]
- Natural diuretic
- Natural antidepressant

Influences that both progestins (synthetic progesterone) and natural progesterone have in common on the body:

- Builds bone[103]
- Helps thyroid hormone function
- Protects against fibrocystic breast disease
- Protects against endometrial cancer
- Normalizes zinc and copper levels

Too much progesterone or progestin can affect weight gain in many ways. Consequences of too much progesterone or progestin:[104,105,106,107,108]

- Increases fat storage
- Decreases glucose tolerance
- Increases risk of insulin resistance by increasing insulin
- Increases appetite
- Increases carbohydrate cravings
- Increases cortisol[109]
- Relaxes the smooth muscles of the gut[110] (can cause bloating, fullness, and constipation)
- Suppresses immune system[111]
- Causes incontinence (leaky bladder)[112]

- Causes ligaments to relax and can cause backaches, leg aches, and achy hips[113]
- Lowers growth hormone[114]

The ratio between estrogen and progesterone also has an effect on ideal body weight. Estradiol lowers body fat by decreasing lipoprotein lipase, an enzyme in the fat cells of the body. Progesterone increases body fat storage by increasing lipoprotein lipase.[115] Furthermore, estrogen and progesterone work together to control the body's release of insulin. Progesterone decreases insulin sensitivity and causes insulin resistance if not in a good ratio with estrogen. Estradiol (E2) increases insulin sensitivity and improves glucose tolerance. Prolonged use of progesterone without adequate estrogen will cause weight gain. It can also cause depression, fatigue, and decreased libido. Too much progesterone in relationship to estrogen can also cause and increase in total cholesterol, LDL (bad cholesterol), and triglycerides, along with a lowering of HDL (good cholesterol).[116] If the estrogen to progesterone ratio is high, it elevates a woman's risk of breast cancer.

Testosterone at menopause and peri-menopause can be normal, low, or high. At menopause, elevated testosterone levels are treated the same way they are if a person has PCOS. Low testosterone levels also affect weight since testosterone increases muscle mass and strength and increases a sense of emotional well-being, self-confidence, and motivation in women.[117] Testosterone also decreases excess body fat and increases muscle tone so that the skin does not sag.[118]

Testosterone also does the following things in the body:

- Increases sexual interest[119]
- Helps maintain memory[120]
- Decreases bone deterioration and helps maintain bone strength[121]

The following are symptoms of testosterone loss:

- Muscle wasting despite adequate calorie and protein intake
- Weight gain and decline in muscle tone
- Fatigue, decreased energy
- Low self-esteem
- Decreased HDL (good cholesterol)[122]
- Decreased sex drive
- Mild depression
- Less dreaming
- Dry, thin skin, with poor elasticity
- Loss of pubic hair
- Thinning and dry hair
- Droopy eyelids
- Sagging cheeks
- Thin lips
- Hypersensitive, hyper-emotional states
- Anxiety

Low testosterone can occur at any age. It may be due to the following:

- Menopause/peri-menopause
- Childbirth
- Chemotherapy
- Surgical menopause[123]
- Adrenal stress or fatigue
- Endometriosis
- Depression
- Psychological trauma
- Birth control pills
- Cholesterol lowering medications called HMG-CoA-reductase inhibitors, such as Lipitor, Mevacor, Zocor, Pravachol, and others are all anti-androgens (will lower testosterone)[124]

What can you do to elevate testosterone levels?

- Decrease calorie intake
- Increase protein in the diet
- Take the amino acids arginine, leucine, glutamine (under a doctor's direction)
- Exercise
- Get enough sleep
- Lose weight
- Practice stress reduction
- Take zinc if you are deficient (Zinc is needed for the metabolism of testosterone.)

Prescription natural testosterone (bio-identical) is the preferred method of testosterone replacement. This would be made by a compounding pharmacy. Methyltestosterone (synthetic) has been suggested to be carcinogenic to the liver (may cause cancer).[125,126,127]

Hormone levels should be measured before any hormonal supplementation is begun. Saliva testing and urine testing are the preferred methods of hormone evaluation for both women and men of all ages. Both methods measure only the "free" form of the hormones. This is important because the free hormone molecules are the only ones that can act directly on the body. Blood levels measure the amount of free and bound hormone. It is also important to measure the hormone levels throughout the entire body. When your healthcare practitioner measures blood levels, only the serum is measured. There are hormones in the red blood cells, which are part of the blood, but this segment is discarded and not measured. Blood levels, furthermore, do not reflect the hormone amounts in all the tissues of the body. As you have seen, there are hormone receptor sites on many different tissues. When saliva or urinary measurements are done, they reflect the levels of hormones throughout the body. I personally use mostly salivary testing since this method allows for the changes of hormone levels over a number of days, as opposed to a one-time blood draw that shows levels only at the time of the test.[128,129,130,131,132,133]

Hormone measurement should be repeated after you begin hormone replacement therapy, usually in about three months. Subsequently, tests should be done on a routine basis depending on your own personal needs. Salivary testing will help your healthcare practitioner better maintain the level of hormone replacement that is right for you.

Male Hormones and Weight Loss

4

For men, DHEA, cortisol, and thyroid hormones have the same effect on weight as for women. Testosterone and estrogen are also involved in how much men will weigh and how easy or difficult it is to lose weight.

Men do go through menopause; it is called andropause. This marks a change in hormonal function with testosterone and DHEA declining and estrogen levels elevating. Half of healthy men between the ages of 50–70 will have a testosterone level below the lowest level seen in healthy men who are 20–40 years of age.[1]

Symptoms of andropause include:[2]

- Weight gain
- Elevated blood sugar
- Fatigue, tiredness, or loss of energy
- Depression, low, or negative mood
- Irritability, anger, or bad temper
- Anxiety or nervousness
- Loss of memory or concentration
- Loss of sex drive or libido
- Loss of erections or problems during sex
- Decreased intensity of orgasms
- Backache, joint pains, or stiffness
- Loss of fitness
- Feeling over-stressed
- Decrease in job performance

- Decline in physical abilities
- Bone loss
- Elevated cholesterol

There are testosterone receptors all over a man's body. Functions of testosterone include:

- Is a sex hormone
- Reduces inflammation[3]
- Involved in the making of protein and muscle formation[4]
- Improves oxygen uptake throughout the body[5,6]
- Helps control blood sugar[7,8]
- Helps regulate cholesterol
- Decreases atherosclerosis (hardening of the arteries)[9,10,11]
- Helps maintain a powerful immune system
- Aids in mental concentration and cognition[12,13,14]
- Improves mood[15]
- Helps protect the brain against Alzheimer's disease[16,17,18]
- Helps manufacture bone[19,20,21]

Testosterone replacement aids all of the above functions (discussed also in the previous references). Replacement is best achieved by having it compounded by a compounding pharmacy. Some drug companies also make testosterone that can be used by men. I usually have it compounded because then the testosterone can be made in the exact dosage that the patient needs. When testosterone is replaced, it helps with weight loss. Testosterone can be given as an injection or by mouth. However, I usually have it given transdermally (on the skin). The reason is that testosterone applied to the skin helps with erectile dysfunction 81% of the time. If it is given orally, it is only 51% effective and if given as injection 53% effective.[22]

An elevation of estrogen levels in a male helps put on weight around the middle. Estrogen elevates as men age due to increased aromatase activity, which is an enzyme that the body produces.

Elevated estrogen levels are also due to alterations in liver function, zinc deficiency, obesity, overuse of alcohol, drug-induced estrogen imbalance, and ingestion of estrogen-containing food or environmental estrogens.[23]

The following medications can elevate estrogen levels in a male. This does not mean that one would stop their medication without discussing it with their doctor first. These medications include:[24]

- Pain/anti-inflammatory drugs:
  NSAIDS (ibuprofen, ketoprofen, and diclofenac), acetaminophen, aspirin
  Propoxeyphene
- Antibiotics: sulfas, tetracyclines, penicillins, cefazolins, erythromycins, floxins, isoniazid
- Antifungal drugs (inhibit P450 systems and act as testosterone receptor inhibitors): miconazole, itraconazole, fluconazole, ketoconazole
- Cholesterol lowering drugs (statins): lovastatin, simvistatin (also decreases testosterone production)
- Antidepressants: fluoxitine, fluvoxamine, paroxetine, sertraline
- Antipsychotic medicines: thorazine, haloperidol
- Heart and blood pressure medicines: propranolol, quinidine, amiodarone (also decreases testosterone production), coumadin, methyldopa
- Antacids: omeprazole, cimetidine
- Vitamins and nutrients: high-dose vitamin E, general dietary deficiencies and malnutrition, grapefruit
- Abusive substances: alcohol, amphetamines, marijuana, cocaine

If a male's estrogen level is high, then it can be lowered by drugs or substances that may speed up the P450 system (see Chapter 8 on detoxification):[25]

- Vitamins: high-dose vitamin C (also increases testosterone production), vitamin K, niacin
- Drugs: phenobarbital, chlordiazepoxide, carbamepazine, trazodone, sulcrafate
- Foods: soy products, vegetarian diets, cruciferous vegetables (broccoli, cauliflower, kale, brussels sprouts), shellfish (oysters), resveratrol

Medications such as chrysin (compounded), progesterone, and Arimidex™ also decrease the amount of estrogen a male makes. Lowering estrogen levels in a male promotes weight loss. It also decreases the risk of heart disease and prostate cancer.

Pregnenolone and Weight Loss

5

Pregnenolone is a precursor to (makes) DHEA, progesterone, estrogen, testosterone, and cortisol in both men and women. Your body synthesizes this hormone from cholesterol. Pregnenolone decreases with age. At age 75, most people have a 65% decline compared to age 35.[1]

Functions of pregnenolone in the body:

- Increases resistance to stress
- Regulates the balance between excitation and inhibition in the nervous system
- Improves energy both physically and mentally
- Enhances nerve transmission and memory
- Reduces pain and inflammation
- Blocks the production of acid-forming compounds

Your natural pathways for producing pregnenolone are blocked when you eat too much saturated fat and trans-fatty acids.[2] Therefore, when you eat the wrong foods, your body does not deal with stress as well, and you do not make the optimum amounts of your other sex hormones. This can cause you to gain weight. Your levels of pregnenolone should be measured and supplemented if you are low. Side effects of overuse of pregnenolone are acne, muscle aches, and drowsiness.

Insulin and Weight Loss

6

Insulin is part of the hormonal symphony in the body that is directly related to weight gain for both women and men.

Estrogen, progesterone, DHEA, testosterone, thyroid hormones, and cortisol are all very important for the regulation of glucose in your body.

Insulin in the body helps regulate glucose, which is your blood sugar. If insulin is not working effectively in your body, this is called insulin resistance. This means that insulin is there, but it is not working as well as it could. Consequently, insulin levels elevate to compensate for their ineffectiveness. There are many causes of high insulin. They include:[1]

- Eating processed high carbohydrate foods
- Increased stress
- Excessive caffeine intake
- Abuse of alcohol
- Nicotine
- Excessive dieting
- Birth control pills or other progestins
- Lack of exercise
- Decreased estrogen (female)
- Increased testosterone (female)
- Decreased testosterone (male)
- Insomnia
- Elevated DHEA
- Hypothyroidism
- Excessive progesterone (female)

Elevated insulin is the common link to obesity, hypertension, and high triglycerides. Insulin increases your ratio of fat to muscle. Consequently, an increase in insulin decreases fat burning.[2] Insulin resistance impairs the body's ability to produce serotonin from tryptophan, which is one of the calming neurotransmitters made by the body (see Chapter 15 on neutrotransmitters).[3]

Symptoms of insulin resistance include:[4]

- Acne
- Ankle swelling
- Burning feet
- Constipation
- Decreased memory or concentration
- Depression
- Fatigue
- Fluctuating high blood pressure
- Fuzzy brain
- Infertility
- Irregular menstrual cycles
- Irritability
- Loose bowel movements alternating with constipation
- Water retention
- Weight gain

When insulin is working in the body, it has other functions besides the regulation of blood sugar. These include:[5]

- Reduces inflammation
- Is anti-thrombotic (reduces blood clots)
- Is an anti-oxidant (decreases oxidation/free radical production)
- Dilates vessels
- Lowers blood pressure
- Decreases atherosclerosis

Treatment is to start with a nutritionally sound eating program. The body needs the following dietary percentages to function optimally:

35% protein
40% carbohydrates
25% good fat

Your brain is 85% fat (yes, we are all fatheads) and is fueled by carbohydrates. Twenty-five percent of the carbohydrates that go into your body go straight to your brain for fueling. If you do not eat enough carbohydrates, then your brain will not have enough fuel for optimal function. It is best to intake low glycemic index foods. These are carbohydrates that do not tend to raise your blood sugar and provide a good source of fuel. The glycemic index (GI) is composed of high glycemic-index foods, moderate glycemic-index foods, and low glycemic-index foods. The glycemic index is a measure of how much a 50 gram portion of a carbohydrate food will raise your blood sugar. Foods higher on the glycemic index raise your blood sugar more and, consequently, elevate insulin levels, which cause you to gain more weight.

High glycemic-index foods:[6]

- Hamburger bun
- New potato
- Semolina
- Shortbread
- Raisins
- Macaroni and cheese, boxed
- Rye flour
- High-fiber crisp rye bread
- Cream of wheat
- Life cereal
- Pineapple
- Carrots
- Angle food cake
- Croissant
- Grape nuts cereal
- Puffed wheat cereal
- Stoned wheat thins
- Soft drinks
- Candy
- English muffin
- Wheat bran, gluten-free
- Shredded wheat cereal
- Melba toast
- Potato, white
- Life savers
- Fruit, dried

(continued)

- Graham crackers
- Bagels
- Watermelon
- Donuts
- Popcorn
- Kaiser rolls
- Corn chips
- Honey
- Cheerios cereal
- French fries
- Pumpkin
- Waffles
- Cocoa puffs cereal
- Rice krispies cereal
- Rice cakes
- Corn chex cereal
- Corn flakes cereal
- Rice
- Rice chex cereal
- Rice pasta, brown
- French baguette
- Tofu frozen desert
- Vanilla wafers
- Broad beans

Moderate glycemic-index foods:[7]

- Macaroni
- Romano beans
- Linguine
- Instant noodles
- Baked beans
- Green peas
- Corn
- Chocolate
- Yams
- Kiwifruit
- Bananas
- Special K cereal
- Buckwheat
- Sweet potatoes
- Potato chips
- Fruit cocktail, canned
- Mango
- Spaghetti, durum
- Orange juice
- Bran chex cereal
- Rice vermicelli
- Blueberry
- Pizza, cheese

Low glycemic-index foods:[8]

- Soybeans
- Rice bran
- Cherries
- Plums
- Barley
- Grapefruit
- Kidney beans
- Peaches
- Lentils
- Green beans
- Black beans
- Apricots
- Lima beans
- Chickpeas
- Rye rice
- Apples
- Pears
- Spaghetti, whole wheat
- Navy beans
- Tomatoes
- Brown beans
- Corn hominy
- All bran cereal
- Black-eyed peas
- Grapes
- Raspberries
- Strawberries
- Blackberries
- Celery
- Peppers
- Mushrooms
- Butterbeans

The glycemic load (GL) is also a measure of carbohydrate content. In other words, how much of the food does it take to increase glucose and insulin. For example, carrots are high on the glycemic index, but it takes a pound a day before blood-sugar and insulin levels elevate. GL = GI divided by 100 times its available carbohydrate content in grams. The glycemic load builds on the GI to provide a measure of total glycemic response to a food. It takes into account a food's GI as well as the amount of carbohydrates per serving. Studies have shown that low glycemic load eating plans have beneficial effects on several obesity-related risk factors compared with a low-fat diet.[9]

Besides a low GI program, the treatment of insulin resistance includes exercise, soluble fiber, and stress reduction. Psychosocial stress can increase glucose and insulin levels.[10,11,12]

Nutrients also help lower blood sugar and make insulin work more effectively in the body. Lentils, chickpeas, and broccoli all decrease insulin levels.

Nutritional treatment of insulin resistance:[13]

- Chromium picolinate 400–600 micrograms
- Lipoic acid 200–600 mg
- CLA 1,000–3,000 mg
- Zinc 25–50 mg
- Vitamin E 600–800 IU
- Taurine 1,000–3,000 mg
- Magnesium 400–800 mg
- Biotin 4–8 mg
- Vanadium 20–50 mg
- Vitamin D 400–2,000 IU
- Coenzyme Q-10 30–200 mg
- B complex 50–100 mg
- Vitamin C 1,000–3,000 mg
- Manganese 5–10 mg
- L-carnitine 250–500 mg
- EPA/DHA 2,000 mg
- Insinase (proprietary neutraceutical by Metagenics, see Appendix)

Herbs can also be used effectively to help manage elevated blood sugar, insulin resistance, and diabetes. Gymnema sylvestre, fenugreek (Trigonella foenum graecum), and bitter gourd (Momordica charantia) have been found to be helpful,[14,15,16,17,18,19,20] as have spices such as cinnamon.[21]

7 Thyroid Hormone Dysfunction and Weight Loss

Thyroid dysfunction can occur at any age. If your level of production of this important hormone is too low, you gain weight. Any imbalance of your thyroid hormone can affect every metabolic function in your body. Your thyroid gland is your body's regulator. It regulates energy and heat production, growth, tissue repair and development, and stimulates protein synthesis. Furthermore, thyroid hormone modulates carbohydrates, protein and fat metabolism, vitamin use, digestion, function of the mitochondria (energy makers of your cells), muscle and nerve action, blood flow, hormone excretion, oxygen utilization, and sexual function to list just some of its uses.

Your body produces more than one kind of thyroid hormone. The main hormones produced by the thyroid gland are T3 and T4. T4 is 80% of the thyroid gland's production. Most of T4 is changed into T3 in your liver or kidneys. T3 is five times more active than T4. T4 can also be converted to reverse T3, which is an inactive form. Your body also makes T2. T2 increases the metabolic rate of your muscles and fat tissue.[1] Decreased T3 production will cause less cholesterol to be removed from your blood, which causes an elevation of LDL (bad cholesterol).[2,3] People with low thyroid levels have cholesterol levels 10–50% higher than people with normal thyroid function.[4] Moreover, mild thyroid dysfunction is associated with heart disease.[5]

T3 is made in other tissues and is called triiodothyronine.

T4 is made in your thyroid gland and is called thyroxine.

TSH (thyroid stimulating hormone) is made in your pituitary gland located in your brain.

The following are symptoms of low thyroid production (hypothyroidism):

- Weight gain
- Depression
- Constipation
- Headaches
- Brittle nails
- Rough, dry skin
- Menstrual irregularities
- Fluid retention
- Poor circulation
- Elbow keratosis
- Diffuse hair loss
- Slow speech
- Anxiety
- Panic attacks
- Decreased memory
- Inability to concentrate
- Muscle and joint pain
- Reduced heart rate
- Slow movements
- Morning stiffness
- Puffy face
- Decreased sexual interest
- Cold intolerance
- Cold hands and feet
- Swollen legs, feet, hands, abdomen
- Insomnia
- Fatigue
- Low body temperature
- Hoarse, husky voice
- Low blood pressure
- Muscle weakness
- Agitation
- Sparse, coarse, dry hair
- Dull facial expression
- Yellowish color of the skin
- Muscle cramps
- Drooping eyelids
- Carpel tunnel syndrome

When your doctor sends you for thyroid studies, your entire thyroid panel should be measured. This includes your TSH, free T3, free T4, reverse T3, and thyroid antibodies. If your antibodies are too high, they can stop thyroid hormone from attaching to your thyroid receptors. Consequently, you can get symptoms of decreased thyroid function even when your blood levels are adequate. Thyroid antibodies can be elevated due to trauma, poor function of your gut, inflammation, and thyroid degeneration.

Many factors affect how your body produces T3 and T4.

Some factors that cause decreased production of T4 include a deficiency in:

- Zinc
- Copper
- Vitamins A, B2, B3, B6, C

Furthermore, your body needs to be able to convert T4 to T3, the more active form. The conversion of T4 to T3 requires an enzyme called 5'diodinase.

Elements that affect 5'diodinase production:[6,7,8,9]

- Selenium deficiency
- Stress
- Cadmium, mercury, or lead toxicity
- Starvation
- Inadequate protein intake
- High carbohydrate diet
- Elevated cortisol
- Chronic illness
- Decreased kidney or liver function

Other factors also cause an inability to convert T4 to T3:[10,11,12]

- Nutrient deficiencies
    - Iodine
    - Iron
    - Selenium
    - Zinc
    - Vitamins A, B2, B6, B12
- Medications
    - Beta blockers
    - Birth control pills[13]
    - Estrogen[14]

  - Lithium
  - Phenytoin
  - Theophylline
  - Chemotherapy
- Diet
  - Cruciferous vegetables (too many)
  - Low protein diet
  - Low fat diet
  - Low carbohydrate diet[15]
  - Excessive alcohol use
  - Soy[16,17]
  - Walnuts
- Other
  - Aging
  - Lipoic acid (too much)
  - Diabetes
  - Fluoride
  - Lead
  - Mercury[18]
  - Pesticides
  - Radiation
  - Stress
  - Surgery
  - Copper excess
  - Calcium excess (You can take too much calcium.)
  - Dioxins
  - PCBs
  - Inadequate production of DHEA, cortisol
  - Phtalates (chemicals added to plastics)

If you cannot convert T4 to T3 adequately, you will have symptoms of thyroid hormone loss. This is also true if you have decreased T3 or increased reverse T3 (stored thyroid hormone).

Factors associated with decreased T3 or increased reverse T3:[19]

- Increased catecholamines (epinephrine, norepinephrine)
- Increased free radical production
- Aging
- Fasting
- Stress
- Prolonged illness
- Diabetes
- Toxic metal exposure
- Elevated IL-6, TNF-alpha, IFN-2 (inflammatory markers)

Furthermore, things that impair your body's response to T3 will cause you to have symptoms of low thyroid. These include iron deficiency and physical inactivity.[20,21]

There are factors that will increase the conversion of T4 to T3 if not enough T3 is being made by your body.

Factors that increase the conversion of T4 to T3:

- Selenium
- Potassium
- Iodine
- Iron
- Zinc
- High protein diet
- Ashwaganda
- Vitamins A, B2, E
- Growth hormone
- Testosterone
- Insulin
- Glucagon
- Melatonin
- Tyrosine

In most cases, it is important that your doctor replace both T3 and T4 if you are diagnosed to have hypothyroidism (low thyroid levels). If you only have your T4 pathway replaced, you may still experience low thyroid symptoms. Replacing T3 and T4 has been found to be more effective than replacing T4 alone.[22] One study revealed that 35% of people on T4 and T3 replacement scored better on mental agility tests. Sixty-seven percent of these people studied state they had an improvement in mood and physical health. Likewise, benefits have been shown by adding T3 for patients already on T4. They have improved mood and brain function.[23]

Synthroid or Levothyroxine are both comprised of only T4. Armour thyroid is T3, T4, and T2 plus other substances that help the body convert T4 to T3 (calcitonin, selenium, and diuretic effect).[24] Some physicians feel that Armour thyroid is not consistent from dose to dose. However, there has never been a complaint to the FDA concerning the inconsistency of Armour thyroid.[25] For a lengthier discussion on thyroid disease, read *Overcoming Thyroid Disorders* by Dr. David Brownstein.[26] Other ways of replacing both thyroid pathways besides taking Armour thyroid is to add T3 (Cytomel) to T4 (Synthroid, etc.). Furthermore, if the ratio of T4 to T3 (4:1) in Armour thyroid is not the correct ratio for you, you could have it compounded by a compounding pharmacy. This is also a prescription. In this way, the ratio between T4 and T3 could be customized to meet your needs.

8 Detoxification and Weight Loss

In order to remain healthy and achieve weight loss, your body has to have the ability to detoxify. Your body has four organs that detoxify. They include: the skin, the kidney, the liver, and the gastrointestinal tract. All of these modalities are modified through environmental exposure, diet, and lifestyle.

Common symptoms of toxin buildup include headaches, muscular aches and pains, and fatigue. Toxicity also can affect your immune, neurological, and endocrine systems.

Immune toxicity may be a factor in asthma, allergies, skin disorders, chronic infections, and cancer.

Neurological toxicity affects cognition, mood, and neurological function.

Endocrine toxicity affects reproduction, menstruation, libido, metabolic rate, stress tolerance, and glucose regulation.

Important facts about your exposure to toxins:

- According to the U.S. Environmental Protection agency, more than 4 billion pounds of chemicals were released into the ground in the year 2000, threatening our natural ground water sources.[1]
- The average American unknowingly eats about 124 pounds of additives a year.[2]
- Each year over 2.5 billion pounds of pesticides are dumped on crop lands, forests, lawns, and fields.[3]

In the environment, you are also exposed to estrogen-like compounds on a routine basis whether you are male or female. These are called xenoestrogens (see Chapter 3: Female Hormones and Weight Loss). They are environmental compounds with estrogenic activity. Xenoestrogens can interfere with or mimic a woman's own hormone synthesis. Xenoestrogens can also raise a male's estrogen level, which increases his risk of prostate cancer and heart disease (see Chapter 4: Male Hormones and Weight Loss). Consequently, xenoestrogens are disruptive to your own hormone production.

Your exposure to toxins is increased by:[4]

- Eating a diet high in processed foods and fat
- Drinking tap water
- Excessive consumption of caffeine containing beverages
- Excessive alcohol consumption
- Tobacco use
- Recreational drug use
- Chronic use of medication(s)
- Lack of exercise
- Liver dysfunction
- Kidney problems
- Intestinal (gut) dysfunction
- Occupational exposure
- Using pesticides, paint, and other toxic substances without adequate protective gear
- Living or working near areas of high vehicle traffic or industrial plants

How Much Toxic Load Are You Carrying?

Detoxification is a process by which your body transforms toxins and medications into harmless molecules that can be eliminated.

The skin is the body's largest absorptive organ. It lets elements in and out of the body in order to maintain hydration and to eliminate toxins.

Your kidney function must be maintained as well if your body wants to detoxify all the additives that are put into it. That is why it is key to drink enough water.

A major part of the detoxification process takes place in the liver. Here, detoxification is largely accomplished in two phases:

Phase I—certain enzymes change toxins into intermediate compounds.

Phase II—other enzymes convert the intermediate compounds created in Phase I into harmless molecules that are eliminated by your body.

Phase I: Your First Line of Defense

In Phase I detoxification, enzymes in the cytochrome P-450 system in the liver use oxygen to modify toxic compounds, medications, and steroid hormones. This is your first line of defense for the detoxification of all environmental toxins, medications, supplements (e.g., vitamins), as well as many waste products that your body produces.

Within your own genetic makeup, there are variations called single nucleotide polymorphisms, called SNPS, pronounced "snips." These SNPs in your genes code for a particular enzyme that can increase or decrease the activity of that enzyme. Both elevated and lowered activity may be harmful to you. Furthermore, if you have increased Phase I clearance without increased Phase II clearance, this can lead to the buildup of intermediate compounds that may be more toxic than the original substance. Decreased Phase I clearance will cause toxic accumulation in your body. Adverse reactions to medications are often due to a decreased capacity for clearing them from your system.

Phase II: Detoxification—Conjugation of Toxins and Elimination

In Phase II detoxification large water-soluble molecules are added to toxins, usually at the reactive site formed by Phase I reactions. After Phase II modifications, the body is able to eliminate the transformed toxins in the urine or the feces.

The completion of the Human Genome Project has made it possible to evaluate genetic variations that affect Phase I and Phase II detoxification and oxidative protection. This genetically-based test is available through Genova Diagnostic Laboratory (see Appendix). Your practitioner, through this kind of testing, can determine whether the detoxification system in your body is working. This allows him or her to identify potential genetic trouble spots in your self-defense system early. Then your clinician can design precise, individualized therapy to support your detoxification. Consequently, many health problems can be avoided and adverse reactions to medications and supplements can be prevented before they happen. For example, one gene evaluated in this profile testing, CYP3A4, affects an enzyme that your body uses to detoxify over 50% of all drugs. These medications include many antidepressants, steroid hormones (like estrogen), and cholesterol-lowering medications. Adverse reactions to prescription drugs have been ranked as the fourth to the sixth leading cause of death in the United States.[5] Each year about 100,000 Americans die from adverse reactions to medications.[6] This is more than double the number killed in motor vehicle accidents.

The detoxification process is very nutrient dependent. Phase I and Phase II enzymes are the engines that drive the detoxification process, and they are fueled by vitamins, minerals, and other key food components. Therefore, if you are undernourished or lack key vitamins or nutrients, you may not be able to deactivate adequately. *Adequate nutrition is essential for effective detoxification.*

Phase I detoxification requires the following nutrients:

- Niacin
- Magnesium
- Copper
- Zinc
- Vitamin C
- Vitamins B2, B3, B6, B12
- Folic acid
- Flavonoids

Phase II detoxification requires the following substances:

- Glutathione
- Vitamin B6
- Glycine
- Taurine
- Glutamine
- Folic acid
- Choline
- Methionine
- Trimethylglycine (TMG)
- S-adenosylmethionine (SAMe)
- Cysteine
- Methionine
- Molybdenum
- Acetyl CoA
- Glucuronic acid

Your body's fourth method of detoxification is your gastrointestinal tract. *You are what you eat.* Your gut is in a constant state of balanced chronic inflammation. This physiologic inflammation is essential for the maturing of the immune system and the development of the normal morphology of the intestinal mucosa. The normal gut flora has 400 different microbial species and numbers more bacteria than there are stars in the sky. The gut has a massive amount of influence on your metabolism. Its metabolic activity is greater than the liver. It has 10 times the number of cells and 100 times the genomic material of other parts of the body. The gastrointestinal tract is also involved with neuroendocrine regulation. Of the body's serotonin, 5% is located in the brain and 95% is located in the gut. If you have any of the following symptoms, your gut is not healthy:

- Nausea
- Belching
- Bloating
- Heartburn
- Abdominal pain

- Cramping
- Abdominal distention
- Depression and anxiety
- Altered bowel function (constipation and/or diarrhea)
- Cramps and spasms
- Hypersecretion of colonic mucus
- Flatulence (gas)
- Halitosis (bad breath)

These are all symptoms of dysbiosis, which is a state of health where the bowel does not function properly. There are also many symptoms that occur outside of the intestinal tract that are linked to dysbiosis. They include:[7]

- Arthralgias (joint pain)
- Anxiety
- Brain fog
- Cognitive and memory deficit
- Depression
- Fatigue
- Fever of unknown origin
- Frequent urination
- Malaise
- Myalgias (muscle aches)
- Palpitations
- Phlebitis
- Pruitis (itching)
- Skin rashes
- Seizures
- Vasculitis (inflammation of vessels)
- Weight gain

There are numerous causes of dysbiosis. Injurious agents such as toxins, alcohol, medications like antibiotics and non-steroidal anti-inflammatory drugs, antacids, poor nutrition (standard American diet), free radical production, stress, diminished HCL (hydrochloric acid), decreased enzymes, diminished bile, food allergies, travel (food, water, bacteria), and high altitudes are also etiologies of dysbiosis.[8]

If the bowel remains unhealthy, then you can get leaky gut syndrome. In this case, the gut allows medications and toxins to leak back into the bloodstream. Weight gain is associated with leaky gut syndrome. When the bowel loses good bacteria, you lose vitamin production and the ability to detoxify adequately and get an overgrowth of harmful species pf gut flora including yeast. Other conditions associated with leaky gut syndrome include:[9]

- Acne
- Aging
- AIDS
- Alcoholism
- Allergies/food sensitivities
- Ankylosing spondylitis
- Arthritis
- Asthma
- Autism
- Burns
- Candida infections
- Celiac disease
- Chemical sensitivities
- Chemotherapy
- Chronic fatigue syndrome
- Crohn's disease
- Cystic fibrosis
- Eczema
- Environmental illness
- Fibromyalgia
- Hyperactivity
- Intestinal infections
- IBS (irritable bowel syndrome)
- Liver dysfunction
- Lupus

- Malabsorption
- Malnutrition
- Psoriasis
- Reiter's syndrome
- Rheumatoid arthritis
- Schizophrenia
- Trauma
- Ulcerative colitis

The evaluation of bowel problems is most comprehensively done by having your practitioner order a comprehensive digestive stool diagnosis (CDSA) (see Appendix for availability). Other studies that may be helpful include a pancreatic elastase test, which reflects overall enzyme production by the gastrointestinal tract including amylase, lipase, and protease. People who most commonly have a deficiency of pancreatic enzymes are ones who have had gallstones or port-cholecystectomy (gallbladder surgical removed) and people over the age of 35 since pancreatic function decreases with age.

The treatment for bowel dysfunction is the 4R program of gut restoration. This includes four components:

Remove
Replace
Repopulate
Restore

The first step is to remove the source of the imbalance. You must then replace with digestive enzymes, hydrochloric acid if needed, and herbal support. Repopulating with lactobacilli, bifidobacteria, and other beneficial bacteria is equally as important. These are called probiotics. Repopulating with prebiotics, which are agents that support the growth and integrity of probiotics, may also be needed. For example, arabinogalactans, active immunoglobulins from whey, lactoferrin, and lactoperoxidase. Likewise, repairing the small bowel with glutamine, gamma oryznol, and glucosamine, or the large bowel with fiber and butyrate has been shown to aid in bowel repair. Boswellia geranium, licorice, quercetin, hydrastis, cheledonium, artemisia, and aloe have all been found to be helpful. Lastly, foods like okra, cabbage, and rice protein along with beneficial fatty acids such as EPA and GLA have all proven to restore health to the gut. A healthy gut makes it easier to lose weight and keep it off.

Having all four methods of detoxification working in the body is required for optimal health and fat burning.

Inflammation and Weight Loss

9

When you are overweight, this sets up an inflammatory response in the body. Inflammation is used by the body to heal, however, when the inflammatory response is too great; then, it can cause disease. Adipose (fat) tissue produces several different "adipokines" including hormones and inflammatory mediators that produce chronic inflammation. One of these adipokines is leptin.

Leptin works on the brain to inhibit food intake and activates thermogenesis (burning of fat) in conjunction with insulin. Fat, fructose, and glucose all lower leptin. Catecholamine production (epinephrine, norepinephrine) also lowers leptin.[1] Methods of raising leptin include weight loss, improvement of insulin function, and improving cholesterol and triglycerides.

Adiponectin is a hormone that the body makes less of if you are overweight. You also make less if you have high insulin, insulin resistance, and/or diabetes. Some of adiponectin's many functions in the body are to lower glucose, improve insulin sensitivity, and promote weight loss. Adiponectin also aids in preventing the transformation of white cells into foam cells, which increase your risk of heart disease and heart attack by narrowing your arteries. Adiponectin is lowered in the body by catecholamines, TNF-alpha, and IL-6 (inflammatory markers).[2]

Acylation stimulating protein (ASP) is produced by adipocytes (fat cells) after interaction in the body with complement C3, factors B and D. ASP increases storage of energy as fat, is elevated after eating, high in overweight people, and is increased by insulin and other things in the body.[3]

Excess adipose tissue is associated with elevated levels of c-reactive protein (CRP), which is a major marker of inflammation. High CRP levels have also been shown to be predictive of the development of type II diabetes.[4] Here, the location of body fat is very predictive. Abdominal fat is more predictive of inflammation levels than other obesity measures.[5]

Adipose tissue is not inactive. It secretes over 50 proteins or adipokines, which have different roles in the body. Adipose tissue may function differently in people who are thin than in people who are overweight. When a person loses weight, his or her inflammatory markers like CRP are lowered.[6]

The glycemic load and glycemic index may play a role in inflammation as well. In a recent medical study of women with diabetes, CRP levels were 32% higher if they were eating a high glycemic index program rather than those eating low glycemic index meals.[7] Another study, this one done on healthy middle-aged women, showed that the glycemic load was significantly related to CRP.[8] High blood sugar and insulin levels are both promoters of inflammation as well.[9]

As previously stated, studies of people who have lost weight revealed a lower CRP and other markers of inflammation.[10,11] In fact, if you get too thin or if you are too heavy, both conditions are associated with increased inflammatory mediators.[12] Physical activity also lowers inflammation.[13]

Chronic psychological stress can also set up an inflammatory response by the body.[14]

Besides weight gain and obesity, inflammation is a symptom of almost every chronic disease process and some acute processes as well. The following are disorders that involve inflammation:[15]

- Arthritis
  - Osteoarthritis
  - Rheumatoid arthritis
  - Gout
- Injuries
  - Tendonitis
  - Bursitis
  - Muscle strains
  - Bruises
- Infections
- Allergies
  - Rhinitis
  - Food allergies
  - Celiac disease/gluten intolerance
- Autoimmune diseases
  - Multiple sclerosis
  - Lupus erythematosus
- Endocrine disorders
  - Diabetes
- Pulmonary
  - Asthma
  - Bronchitis
  - Chronic obstructive pulmonary disease (COPD)
- Cardiovascular
  - Coronary artery disease
  - Myocarditis
  - Hypertension
- Cancer
  - Lung
  - Breast
  - Prostate
  - Gastric
- Neurological
  - Alzheimer's disease

- Skin
  - Sunburn
  - Eczema and dermatitis
  - Psoriasis
- Dental
  - Gingivitis
  - Periodontitis
- Eye
  - Conjunctivitis
  - Uveitis
- Digestive tract
  - Gastritis, ulcers
  - Crohn's disease
  - Ulcerative colitis
  - Diverticulitis
  - Irritable bowel syndrome (IBS)

Your body requires fats to decrease inflammation, to prevent disease, and to make your body work. The major recent shift in food consumption to a low-fat diet deprives your body of essential fatty acids. Instead of eliminating fat from your diet, you need to add "good" fats to your eating and nutrient supplementation program.

Functions of fatty acids in your body:[16,17,18,19,20]

- Decreases inflammation
- Enhances insulin action
- Provides structural support for the outer walls or membranes of the body's cells
- Helps convert the nutrients from foods into useable forms of energy
- Involved in cell to cell communication

- Makes it possible for nutrients to pass from the blood through the cell walls
- Helps with substances in the cells to pass into the blood
- Used to manufacture red blood cells
- Dilates or constricts blood vessels in the stomach, intestines, uterus, and bronchial tree
- Lowers triglycerides
- Makes blood less sticky
- Raises HDL (good cholesterol)
- Decreases arrhythmias (irregular heart rhythm)
- Lowers blood pressure
- May decrease homocysteine levels
- Helps protect against oxidation and ischemic heart disease
- Needed for normal development and function of your brain, eyes, inner ear, adrenal glands, and reproductive tract
- Needed to make prostaglandins I and III which decrease inflammation, increase in immune function, and decrease menstrual cramps
- Reduces PMS symptoms
- Important for mitochondrial function (energy producing parts of your body)

Fats occur in the following groups:

- Supersaturated/Omega-3 fatty acids
- Polyunsaturated/Omega-6 fatty acids
- Monounsatured/Omega-9 fatty acids
- Monounsaturated/Omega-7 fatty acids
- Saturated fatty acids

The omega-6 fatty acids produce inflammation, and the omega-3 fatty acids decrease inflammation.[21]

Omega-3 fatty acids:

- Alpha-linolenic acid, which is in flax, hemp seed, canola, soy bean, walnut, and dark green leaves
- Stearidonic acid occurs in black currant seeds
- Eicosapentaenoic acid (EPA) and docosahexaenoic acid (DHA) occur in fish, nuts, and lamb

Omega-6 fatty acids occur in:

- Linoleic acid occurs in safflower, sunflower, hemp, soybean, walnut, pumpkin, sesame, and flax oil
- Gamma-linolenic acid (GLA) occurs in borage oil, black current seed, and evening primrose oil
- Dihumogamma-linolenic acid (DGLA) occurs in mother's milk
- Arachidonic acid occurs in meats and animal products

The following are clinical manifestations of essential fatty acid deficiency:[22,23]

- Weight gain
- Dry, scaly skin/dermatitis
- Dry hair, dandruff
- Brittle nails, graying with horizontal splitting
- Thirst, excessive urination
- Decreased memory and mental abilities
- Psychological disturbances
- Impaired immune response
- Fatty infiltration of the liver
- Tingling or numbness of your arms or legs (neuropathy)
- Reduced vision
- Increased cholesterol
- Mood swings
- Depression

- Age-related memory decline
- Arthritis
- Asthma
- Slow wound healing
- Sterility in men
- Miscarriage
- Heart disease
- Hair loss
- Cracking skin at finger tips
- Bumps on back of arms

There are two essential fats that your body cannot make by itself and so you have to ingest them. They are linoleic acid (omega-6 fatty acid) and linolenic acid (omega-3 fatty acid). Neither of these groups of fatty acids can be made by your body, and therefore they must be eaten or taken as a supplement.

Your body requires omega-6 fatty acids to maintain your health. However, if you intake too many of them, you cause inflammation by producing prostaglandins that go down an inflammatory pathway instead of an anti-inflammatory pathway. The standard American diet is very low in omega-3 fatty acids and very high in omega-6 fatty acids. It is best to intake three to six parts of omega-6 fatty acids to one part omega-3 fatty acids instead of what most American eat, which is between 10:1 and 25:1. This is why the standard American diet is abbreviated SAD because it is truly sad.

Your body requires zinc, magnesium, niacin, vitamin C, vitamin A, biotin, B vitamins, and other nutrients to convert fatty acids.[24]

There are many things that cause a deficiency of fatty acids in your body. An increase in sugar intake will interfere with the enzymes needed to make fatty acids. Other reasons for fatty acid deficiency include:[25]

- Decreased intake of the right kind of fatty acids
- Stress
- Inability to absorb fatty acids

- Alcoholism
- Type I diabetes
- Decreased intake of nutrients needed as cofactors
- Carnitine deficiency
- Increase in trans-fatty acid intake (interferes with fatty acid synthesis)

Trans-fatty acids do not occur naturally. They were developed by the food industry to help food stay fresh longer. They have been shown to increase LDL (bad cholesterol), lower HDL (good cholesterol), increase triglycerides, increase lipoprotein (a) (a major risk factor for heart disease), and make platelets stickier, which increases blood clots. Furthermore, trans-fatty acids cause your cell membranes to leak, disrupting cellular metabolism and allowing toxins to enter your cells.[26] All processed oils contain trans-fatty acids. Consequently, it is best to avoid processed oils. The more solid the oil, the more trans-fatty acids are included in it. Liquid vegetable oils contain up to 6% trans-fats and margarines and shortening up to 58% trans-fatty acids.[27] In Europe, there are mandates against trans-fatty acids. Recently, the city of New York has looked at banning trans-fatty acids as well. The restaurant industry is now also changing the way it does business, with Denny's restaurants announcing plans to remove trans-fats from their menu. Anything that says hydrogenated or partially hydrogenated contains trans-fatty acids. Trans-fatty acids will increase your risk of heart disease. Furthermore, trans-fatty acids interfere with your body's ability to make its own DHA.[28]

Trans-fatty acids occur in:

- Boxed foods
- Breads
- Candies
- Chocolate
- Frozen diners
- Processed meats
- French fries
- Potato chips
- Corn chips/tortilla chips
- Donuts
- Pastries
- Margarine
- Mayonnaise

Fatty acid intake can decrease inflammation and therefore make weight loss easier. Fatty acids may also change the amount of medication that you may need. You may require less Prozac or insulin, for example.[29] If you are taking blood thinners, then consult your doctor concerning the amount of fatty acids you should take.

Fatty acids can become rancid and therefore should be refrigerated. If you take natural vitamin E when using omega-3-fatty acids, it helps prevent oxidation. Some people experience burping up of fatty acids. This can be avoided by putting them in the freezer prior to use. This does not destroy their effectiveness. Have your doctor measure your essential and metabolic fatty acids. See Appendix for availability.

The Mediterranean diet lowers inflammation. A recent medical study showed that one meal of the Mediterranean style could lower CRP whereas the standard American diet could not.[30] Longer studies have revealed the same thing.[31] As discussed previously in this chapter, weight loss is associated with a decrease in inflammatory markers IL-1, IL-18, TNF-alpha, and CRP.[32]

The following nutrients will all work for inflammation. They are grouped according to classifications.

Agents to decrease inflammation:[33]

- Essential fatty acids
  - EPA
  - GLA
- Niacinamide
- Pantothenic acid
- Proteases (bromelain)
- Glucosamine
- Bioflavonoids
  - Quercetin
  - Grape seed extract and pycnogenol
  - Hesperidin
- Antioxidants

Plant pigments with antioxidant properties:[34]

- Carotenoids (lycopene, beta carotene)
- Green tea catechins (polyphenols)
- Anthocyanidins (beets, berries, grapes)
- Quercetin (fruits and vegetable rind)
- Curcuminoids (turmeric)
- Trans-resveratrol (a phytoalexin from grapes)

Potent herbal antioxidants:[35]

- Ashwaganda (*Withania somnifera*)
- Blueberry/bilberry (*Vaccinium myrtillus*)
- Chocolate (*Theobroma cacao*)
- Cranberry (*Vaccinium macrocarpon*)
- Garlic (*Allium sativum*)
- Ginkgo (*Gingko biloba*) Do not take with coumadin or other blood thinners.
- Ginger (*Zingiber officinalis*) Do not take with coumadin or non-steroidal anti-inflammatory medications.
- Green tea (*Camellia sinensis*)
- Grape seed (*Vitus vinifera*)
- Hawthorne (*Crataegus oxyacantha*)
- Horse chestnut (*Aesculus hippocastanum*)
- Milk thistle (*Silybum marianum*)
- Oregano (*Origanum vulgare*)
- Purple grape (*Vitis labrusca*)
- Rosemary (*Rosmarinus officinalis*)
- Turmeric (*Curcuma longa*)

Botanicals found to have anti-inflammatory properties:[36]

- Willow bark (*Salix species*)
- Licorice root (*Glycyrrhiza glabra*)
- Boswellia (*Boswellia serrata*)
- Bromelain (*Ananus comosus*)
- Chinese skullcap (*Scutellaria baicalensis*)
- Turmeric (*Curcuma longa*)

- Ginger (*Zingiber officinalis*) Do not take with coumadin or non-steroidal anti-inflammatory medications.
- Cayenne pepper (*Capsicum annuum*)
- Aloe vera (*Aloe barbadensis*)
- Green tea (*Camellia sinensis*)
- Ginkgo (*Ginkgo biloba*) Do not take with coumadin or other blood thinners.

Natural COX-2 inhibitors:[37]

- Bromelain (pineapple stem: *Ananus comosus*)
- Capsaicin (cayenne: *Capsicum annuum*)
- Carnosol and carnosic acid (rosemary)
- Carvacrol (oregano: *Oreganum vulgare*)
- Chinese skullcap (*Scutellaria baicalensis*)
- Curcumin (turmeric: *Curcuma longa*) Do not take with non-steroidal anti-inflammatory medications.
- Feverfew (*Tanacetum parthenium*)
- Gamma tocopherol
- Gingerol/shogaol (ginger: *Zingiber officinalis*)
- Green tea catechins (*Camellia sinensis*)
- Melatonin
- Trans-resveratrol (purple grape)
- Thymol (thyme: *Thymus bulgaris*)
- Quercetin
- Willow bark (*Salix species*)

See the Appendix for list of some of the neutraceutical companies that your practitioner can use to treat chronic inflammation.

Nutritional requirements are also affected by the production of free radicals. Your body creates free radicals in many of the reactions that occur to produce energy and other substances. Free radicals are molecules that lack an electron. They will eventually rob your cells of electrons that cause damage and contribute to oxidative stress, which accelerates aging and leads to disease. Therefore, free radical production can cause weight gain since it sets up an inflammatory response. In today's world, free radicals occur in the environment as well.

Causes of free radical production outside of the body:

- Television screens
- Cell phones (electromagnetic fields)
- Computer screens
- Airplane trips
- Hair dryers
- Fluorescent lights
- Microwaving
- Toxic exposure to chemicals in your food, water, and air
- Excessive sunlight

When you have exposure to free radicals in the environment, your body cannot handle this extra load of oxidation. Oxidation in your body is like rust on your car. If you have extra free radicals bombarding your body all day long, your system will "rust" on the inside. Cataract formation is an example of this. In order to stop the oxidative process, you can take antioxidants, which donate an electron to the free radical. This stops the destructive course.

The following is a list of some of the antioxidants that you can take:

- Vitamin A
- Vitamin C
- Vitamin E
- Selenium
- Coenzyme Q-10
- Alpha lipoic acid
- Melatonin
- Garlic
- Glutathione/NAC

Furthermore, it is paramount that antioxidants be balanced. In certain conditions, too much of one antioxidant may stop the protective affects of other antioxidants.[39,40] Stress also depletes your body of vitamins and minerals, including antioxidants. Likewise, as you age, you need more nutrients. For example, as you grow older, your body makes less alpha lipoic acid and less coenzyme Q-10.

Sleep Deprivation and Weight Loss

10

Adequate sleep is needed to maintain health and to promote weight loss. Ineffective sleep elevates inflammatory markers in the body such as IL-6 and your stress hormone cortisol.[1,2] Studies have shown that people who get less than six and one-half hours of sleep a night for eight consecutive nights have less insulin sensitivity than those who sleep seven to eight hours a night.[3] Therefore, insulin will not work as effectively in the body, and you can gain weight and predispose yourself to diabetes by not having adequate sleep. Chronic partial sleep is also associated with decreased leptin levels.[4]

Approximately 60 million Americans a year have some sort of insomnia.[5] This includes having trouble falling asleep, awakening several times during the night, waking up too early in the morning, and not feeling refreshed upon awakening. Sleep is paramount in keeping healthy. When you sleep is when your body repairs and also makes growth hormone (the hormone that keeps you younger).[6]

Consequently, the metabolic consequences of disturbed sleep include:[7]

- Weight gain
- Increased stress hormone
- Elevated inflammatory markers
- Increased risk for abnormal insulin level and function
- Increased cardiovascular risk

- Increased fatigue
- Short-term memory loss
- Disruption of thyroid metabolism
- Alteration in leptin relationships
- Lowered growth hormone production

A medical study revealed the following results of sleep deficit in young adults:[8]

- 40% longer to regulate blood sugar than normal to process a high carbohydrate meal
- Insulin secretion and response to insulin decreased
- TSH (thyroid stimulating hormone) secretion down
- Cortisol increased

This study revealed that the consequences of sleep deprivation mimic the effects of aging and early diabetes. Insomnia is related in many cases to neurotransmitter dysfunction. Serotonin, dopamine, and methylation of other catecholamines are involved. Therefore, you may want to have your neurotransmitter levels measured (see Chapter 15 on neurotransmitters) along with your melatonin levels (see Appendix for availability).

Factors that contribute to insomnia:[9,10,11]

- Diet
  - Caffeinated beverages
  - Food allergies
  - Food additives
- Illness
  - Urinary disorders
  - Nasal and sinus problems
  - Hiatal hernia/reflux esophagitis
  - Anxiety disorder
  - Depression
  - Asthma

Gallbladder disease
Chronic pain

- Hormonal
  - Thyroid dysfunction
  - Growth hormone loss
  - Progesterone loss (women)
  - Testosterone loss (men)
  - Estrogen loss (women)
  - Elevated cortisol
- Medications
  - Asthma medications
  - Sleeping pills
  - Blood pressure medications
  - Synthetic progestins
- Exercise (lack of)
- Sleep apnea
- Light
- Shift work
- Nutritional deficiency
  - Niacin deficiency
  - Magnesium deficiency
  - Copper deficiency or excess
  - Low iron
  - Tryptophan deficiency
  - Vitamin B6 deficiency
- Chemical exposure (over 100 chemicals can decrease sleep)

If you have insomnia, melatonin levels should be measured. One of the most accurate methods of measuring melatonin is by saliva testing. This way, you can measure melatonin several times during the day and at 3 o'clock A.M. to aid in better determining your need for melatonin replacement.[12] Melatonin is another hormone that your body makes. It sets your body's 24-hour cycle. Melatonin is made from the amino acid tryptophan, which is also used to make serotonin. Therefore, when melatonin goes up, serotonin goes down. If you eat too many high-sugar carbohydrates, you will make less melatonin because carbohydrates shift your amino acid balance to make more serotonin.[13]

You need B vitamins to convert melatonin from tryptophan. Therefore, if you do not have an adequate intake of vitamin B rich foods or do not take a supplement, your body may be deficient in melatonin.

Melatonin influences the following:[14,15,16,17]

- Sleep
- Mood
- Stress response
- Immune function
- Release of sex hormones
- Antioxidant activity (more potent than vitamin C or E)[18, 19, 20]
- Helps to prevent cancer
- Blocks estrogen from binding to estrogen receptors[21]
- Stimulates the parathyroid gland, which regulates bone formation[22]
- Stimulates the production of growth hormone
- Decreases cortisol
- Increases the action of benzodiazepine medications

Factors that can decrease melatonin:[23, 24]

- Beta blockers
- Calcium channel blockers
- Alpha adrenergic blockers
- Ibuprofen
- Tranquilizers
- Aspirin
- Caffeine
- Alcohol
- Tobacco
- Electromagnetic fields[25]

Supplementation, sleep, and exercise increase melatonin production.[26]

Like any hormone, you can have too much melatonin.

Side effects of too much melatonin:

- Elevates cortisol, which can increase fat storage[27]
- Suppresses serotonin, which will increase your carbohydrate cravings
- Intense dreaming, nightmares
- Daytime sleepiness/fatigue
- Depression
- Headaches

If you supplement with too much melatonin, you may suppress estrogen and testosterone in the body if you are a woman. In contrast, if you have too little melatonin, you may increase the risk of age-related diseases if you are male or female.[28] Consequently, it is very important to have the right amount of this hormone in your body.

Supplements for insomnia:[29,30,31,32,33,34,35,36]

- Magnesium 600 mg
- GABA 300–900 mg
- 5-HTP 100–200 mg
- Inositol 1,000 mg
- Melatonin 1–6 mg
- Lemon balm (cannot use if pregnant or have glaucoma)
- Passion flower (cannot take if on MAO inhibitor or pregnant)
- Jujube (cannot take if pregnant)
- Astragalus (cannot take if gum allergy)
- Camomile (may have allergy to if allergic to ragweed)

Exercise and Weight Loss

11

In order to lose weight and keep it off, exercise is a key element.

Researchers at Princeton determined that exercise is important for weight loss due to the following reasons:[1,2,3,4,5,6,7]

- Aids in increasing metabolic rate
- Increases activation of brown fat, which burns fat (white adipose tissue stores fat)
- Elevates activation of the sympathetic nervous system, which aids in burning fat
- Increases growth hormone release, which aids in weight loss and keeping the body younger
- Improves the sensitivity of insulin
- Helps fat loss while maintaining lean muscle

Fiber Intake and Weight Loss

12

An adequate intake of fiber is important for weight loss because it improves digestive health and makes you feel full. Fiber also helps keep your blood sugar stable, which helps insulin work more effectively.[1] It has no caloric value, so you do not gain weight when you ingest fiber. The optimal intake is between 30 and 50 grams of fiber a day. Most Americans intake approximately 15 grams of fiber on a daily basis.

There are two types of fiber, soluble and insoluble. Soluble fiber lowers cholesterol, reduces blood sugar, lowers blood pressure, and promotes growth of good bacteria.[2,3,4,5,6] Pectins, gums, and mucilages fall into this category. Insoluble fibers include cellulose, lignins, and hemicellulose. This kind of fiber aids in digestion and waste elimination. It also promotes bowel regularity and has a cleansing effect.

Sources of soluble fiber:[7,8]

- Apples
- Apricots
- Bananas
- Chick peas
- Oat bran
- Broccoli
- Psyllium
- Barley
- Cabbage
- Flax seed
- Nuts
- Okra
- Oranges
- Grapefruit
- Pears
- Pinto, navy, lima, and kidney beans
- Prunes
- Split peas
- Sweet potatoes

Insoluble fiber sources:[9,10]

- Grains
- Beans
- Celery
- Corn
- Lentils
- High-fiber cereal
- Potato (with skin)
- Wheat bran
- Prunes
- Bananas
- Broccoli
- Brown rice
- Brussels sprouts
- Cauliflower
- Spinach
- Wheat bran (unprocessed)
- Whole wheat bread
- Pasta
- Crackers

13

Water and Weight Loss

Drinking enough water helps the body feel full and decreases your intake of additional calories. The amount of water you need in one day is: one-half your body weight in ounces.[1] For example, if you weigh 200 pounds, then you need to drink 100 ounces of water a day. Other forms of liquid *cannot* be included in this. Some beverage forms have the opposite effect and dehydrate you like coffee and tea.

Water that you drink should be purified. Steam distilled is the best. With steam distilled water, however, all of the minerals are removed, and you will need to get them from your food or replace them with vitamin intake.

14 Yeast Infections and Weight Loss

You may have a difficult time staying away from sugar if you have chronic yeast infections. *Candida albicans* is a yeast organism that occurs in the body, but if it is allowed to over-flourish and dominate the intestinal flora, it can become pathologic. Yeast overgrowth can result in leaky gut syndrome. I have found that when I treat a patient's chronic yeast infection that it is much easier for him or her to lose weight.

A great book on this subject is *The Yeast Connection Handbook* by William Crook.[1] Nancy Appleton in her book, *Stopping Inflammation*, also has a great chapter on yeast.[2]

Symptoms of yeast infections:[3,4]

- Allergic and Upper Respiratory
  - Asthma
  - Blurred vision
  - Body aches and tension
  - Bronchitis (recurrent)
  - Burning or tingling
  - Headaches
  - Nasal congestion
  - Numbness
  - Chemical sensitivity
  - Chest pain
  - Coughing
  - Earaches

  - Hay fever
  - Painful, swollen, stiff joints
  - Shortness of breath
  - Sinusitis
  - Sore throat
  - Uticaria (hives, wheals or welts)
- Cognitive
  - Attention deficit disorder (ADD)/ADHD
  - Confusion
  - Disorientation
  - Drowsiness
  - Fatigue
  - Feelings of unreality
  - Hyperactivity
  - Inability to concentrate
  - Poor memory
- Emotional
  - Anxiety
  - Depression
  - Irritability
  - Mood swings
  - Nervousness
  - Obsessive-compulsive disorder
- Gastrointestinal
  - Bloating
  - Constipation
  - Crohn's disease
  - Diarrhea
  - Dry mouth
  - Gas
  - Halitosis (bad breath)
  - Heartburn
  - Indigestion
  - Inflammation
  - Irritable bowel syndrome (IBS)

Lactose intolerance
Oral thrush
Rectal itching

- Genitourinary
  - Bladder infection (recurrent)
  - Burning on urination
  - Cystitis (bladder inflammation)
  - Fluid retention
  - Frequent urination
  - Impotency
  - Infertility
  - Loss of sexual feelings
  - Prostatitis
- Glandular and Autoimmune
  - Adrenal dysfunction
  - Cold hands or feet
  - Diabetes mellitus
  - Hypoglycemia
  - Hypothyroidism
  - Low body temperature
  - Lupus erythematosus
  - Multiple sclerosis
  - Rheumatoid arthritis
  - Scleroderma
- Skin
  - Acne
  - Athlete's foot
  - Dandruff
  - Diaper rash
  - Dry skin
  - Eczema
  - Excessive perspiration
  - Facial rash
  - Fungus infection of the nails
  - Impetigo (skin infection)

Inflammation of hair follicles
Psoriasis
Seborrheic dermatitis
Tinea cruris (jock itch)

- Women's Issues
    Cramps
    Endometriosis
    Menstrual irregularities
    Painful intercourse
    Premenstrual syndrome (PMS)
    Recurrent yeast vaginitis
    Vaginal burning, itching or discharge
    Vulvodynia (vulvar burning)

There are other complaints and illnesses found in adults that may be yeast-related that are not obvious. One of the most common is chronic sinusitis. One study showed positive fungal cultures in nasal secretions of 96% of 210 consecutive chronic sinusitis patients.[5] Other illnesses and complaints include:[6]

- Chronic fatigue syndrome
- Fibromyalgia
- Myasthenia gravis
- Tingling

There are many causes of yeast infection. Overuse of antibiotics is one of the most common. Also, if you have an elevated blood sugar or other reason to be immunocompromised, it increases your risk of developing a yeast infection. Other etiologies of yeast infections include: hormonal changes associated with the normal menstrual cycle, birth control pill use, pregnancy, steroid use, genital irritations and abrasions, alcohol, antacids, chemicals and toxins, chemotherapy, chronic constipation or diarrhea, diabetes, diets high in sugar, excessive stress, intestinal parasites, steroid use, thyroid disease, and re-infection from your sexual partner.[7,8]

Diagnosis of chronic yeast infections can be done by having your doctor order a blood study for candida immune complex assay, which is a blood test that detects the presence of antibodies to yeast, or you can see a fellowship trained anti-aging and functional medicine practitioner and have a comprehensive digestive stool analysis done (see Appendix for availability). Treatment usually includes a prescription anti-fungal agent to be taken for two months. It is also important to take probiotics (live bacteria) to repopulate the gut for at least six months to a year. Nonprescription anti-yeast and herbal treatments of yeast infections are also very helpful, including caprylic acid, citrus seed extract, garlic, tanalbit, tricycline (grapefruit seed extract, artemesia, and berberine), paracan (black walnut hulls, wormwood, pumpkin seed, pau d'arco, echinacea, barberry, gentian, garlic, olive leaf, cloves, chamomile, and thyme), goldenseal, aloe vera, and colloidal silver.[9] Eliminating sugar from your diet along with packaged and processed foods will help speed your recovery. Avoiding foods that contain fungi or molds is also helpful:[10]

- Breads, pastries, and other raised bakery goods
- Cheeses
- Condiment, sauces, and vinegar-containing foods (use freshly squeezed lemon juice in salad dressings)
- Malt products
- Processed and smoked meats
- Edible fungi (mushrooms, morels, and truffles)
- Melons
- Dried and candied fruits
- Leftovers

Dr. Crook's recommended supplements for people with yeast-related health problems:[11]

• Vitamin A	5,000–10,000 IU
• Beta-carotene	15,000 IU
• Vitamin B1	25–100 mg

- Vitamin B2 50 mg
- Niacin 50 mg
- Niacinamide 100–150 mg
- Pantothenic acid 100–500 mg
- Vitamin B6 25–100 mg
- Folic acid 200–800 micrograms
- Vitamin B12 100–2,000 mg
- Biotin 300 micrograms
- Choline 100 mg
- Vitamin C 1,000–10,000 mg
- Vitamin D 100–400 IU
- Vitamin E 400–600 IU
- Calcium 500 mg
- Magnesium 500 mg
- Inositol 100 mg
- Citrus bioflavonoids 100 mg
- PABA 50 mg
- Zinc 15–30 mg
- Copper 1–2 mg
- Manganese 5–20 mg
- Selenium 100–200 micrograms
- Chromium 200 micrograms
- Molybdenum 100 micrograms
- Vanadium 25 micrograms
- Boron 1 mg

Neurotransmitters and Weight Loss 15

Neurotransmitters are the chemical messengers that relay signals between nerve cells and are present throughout the body. Symptoms of neurotransmitter dysfunction include:[1]

- Fatigue
- Chronic muscle and joint pain
- Inappropriate hunger or food cravings
- Irritability
- Hostility
- Inability to concentrate or focus
- Agitation
- Depression
- Excessive body fat
- Obsessive/compulsive behaviors
- Sleep disturbances
- Stress symptoms
- Recurrent diarrhea/constipation
- Headaches/migraines

Weight gain and obesity for many people can be related to neurotransmitter dysfunction. There are many other clinical conditions related to neurotransmitter imbalances. They include:[2]

- Inappropriate stress reaction
- Depression
- Migraine

- Anxiety
- Insomnia
- Irritable bowel syndrome (IBS)
- ADD/ADHD
- Hypertension
- Fibromyalgia
- Chronic fatigue

Neurotransmitter dysfunction may also be associated with trauma, hypoxia (loss of oxygen), hypoglycemia (low blood sugar), Huntington's disease, Parkinson's disease, Alzheimer's disease, vascular dementia, amyotrophic lateral sclerosis (ALS), Tourette's syndrome, and Korsakoff's syndrome.[3]

There are two kinds of neurotransmitters in the body. They are inhibitory and excitatory neurotransmitters. The brain depends on a delicate balance of excitatory and inhibitory systems.

Inhibitory neurotransmitters decrease the ability to send signals and have a calming effect on the body. They include GABA, serotonin, glycine, taurine, and agmatine.

GABA is an inhibitory neurotransmitter of the brain that occurs in 30–40% of all nerve endings. These nerve endings are called synapses. GABA is found in large amounts in the area of the brain known as the hypothalamus. GABA is made from glutamine, which is an amino acid in the body (see below). It requires pyridoxal 5'phosphate as a cofactor. GABA forms a chloride ion channel in the cell. This is how barbiturates and alcohol affect the GABA receptor as well. When you take GABA, it is important that the vitamin B6 also be taken to act as a cofactor. Otherwise, the body cannot metabolize GABA properly.

Functions of GABA:[4,5,6]

- Is an inhibitory neurotransmitter
- Produces a calming effect on the brain
- Aids secreting growth hormone
- Muscle relaxant

- Lowers blood pressure
- Helps control hypoglycemia
- Prevents anxiety
- Promotes sleep

Symptoms of GABA deficiency:[7]

- Anxiety
- Sensation that the brain is racing out of control

Foods that contain GABA are beans, brewer's yeast, dairy products, eggs, fish, legumes, meat, nuts, seafood, seeds, soy, whey, and whole grains.[8] GABA is not without side effects. Some people experience a tingling sensation in the face and a slight shortness of breath after taking GABA, which usually lasts for only a few minutes. It may make you drowsy, so it is suggested that you take GABA in the evening. GABA should not be taken if you have kidney or liver disease, and consultation with a physician is always recommended before taking GABA.

Dosage:

Weight less than 125 pounds, 375 mg three times a day
Weight more than 125 pounds, 750 mg three times a day

Serotonin is an inhibitory neurotransmitter and is made from tryptophan and 5-HTP. It is present in the brain, platelets, retina, and in the gastrointestinal tract. The highest concentrations are found in the gut and platelets. After release from the neurons, most of the released serotonin is recaptured (re-uptaked). Tryptophan and 5-HTP are used to treat weight gain, depression, compulsive disorders, anxiety, and migraines. They decrease the stress response.[9,10]

Tryptophan works best if it is taken with B6 and carbohydrates. The body requires B6 to make tryptophan. It is available with and without a prescription in the United States.

Functions of tryptophan:[11,12,13]

- Makes serotonin
- Acts as a mood stabilizer
- Helps with insomnia
- Increases the release of growth hormone
- Suppresses appetite
- Needed for the production of vitamin B3

Foods that contain tryptophan are turkey, chicken, pork, fish, beans, dairy products, eggs, grains, cereals, nuts, and seeds. If you are taking a SSRIs or MAO inhibitors for depression, you should not take tryptophan.

Dosage: 5–50 mg

5-HTP (5-hydroxytryptophan) manufactures serotonin. It is used to treat weight gain, carbohydrate cravings, stress, depression, fibromyalgia, chronic headaches, insomnia, hyperactivity, PMS, obsessive-compulsive disorder, addiction, anxiety, and pain.[14,15,16,17,18] If you are taking an SSRI or other antidepressant, then it is contraindicated to take 5-HTP. Magnesium prolongs the benefits of 5-HTP administration.

Dosage: 50–300 mg

Having a normal serotonin level is key to sticking to a healthy eating program. Low serotonin increases the likelihood of you eating junk food. Having a high serotonin helps you with not craving sweets even if they are placed in front of you. Stress depletes the body of serotonin. Other ways to elevate serotonin besides 5-HTP and tryptophan are the use of whey protein, phosphtidylserine, omega-3-fatty acids, and inositol.

Glycine is another inhibitory neurotransmitter. It is an amino acid and has many other functions in the body, including:[19,20]

- Decreases sugar cravings
- Important in the manufacture of glucose from glycogen in the liver
- Used in the synthesis of hemoglobin, glutathione, DNA, and RNA
- Needed to maintain the nervous system
- Needed for prostate gland function
- Helps form collagen
- Involved in the metabolism of bile salts
- Helps detoxify heavy metals from the body
- Calms aggression
- Used in metabolism of proteins

Glycine is naturally found in meats and wheat germ.[21] If you are taking clozapine or a related medication, you should not take glycine.[22]

Dosage: 500–3,000 mg

Likewise, taurine is an inhibitory neurotransmitter and requires zinc to help it function properly. In an adult, taurine is made from methionine and cysteine. When you are stressed, the body becomes depleted of taurine. In children, taurine is an essential amino acid, which means that it must be taken in. Like the other inhibitory neurotransmitters, taurine has numerous functions in the body.

Functions of taurine:[23,24,25,26,27,28,29]

- Aids in glucose metabolism by increasing the activity of insulin receptors
- Improves insulin sensitivity
- Is a natural diuretic
- Improves lung health
- Protects cell membranes from damage
- Detoxifies toxic substances

- Needed for kidney function
- Helps modulate calcium movement
- Required for the formation of bile salts
- Lowers blood pressure
- Boosts antioxidant defense
- Supports immune function
- Strengthens the heart muscle
- Stabilizes heart rhythm
- Prevents blood clots
- Aids wound healing
- Improves fat metabolism in the liver

Symptoms of taurine deficiency include anxiety, seizure, hyperactivity, and impaired brain function.[30] Taurine is used in the treatment of weight loss, diabetes, macular degeneration, epilepsy, congestive heart failure, high blood pressure, heart disease, iron deficiency anemia, psoriasis, wound healing, and is helpful to decrease the side effects of radiation and chemotherapy.[31,32,33,34,35,36,37,38,39,40] A few foods contain taurine, including brewer's yeast, dairy products, eggs, fish, meat, and seafood. It should not be taken with aspirin or any other salicylate. If the body's homocysteine level is high, there may be a block in the pathway that makes taurine.

Dosage: 1–4 grams. The requirement for taurine increases when you are stressed or ill.

The last inhibitory neurotransmitter that is going to be discussed is agmatine, which modulates the actions of glutamate. It is a metabolite of arginine. Arginine promotes many functions in the body, including:[41,42,43,44,45]

- Needed for secretion of glucagon and insulin
- Increases immune function by increasing natural killer cell activity
- Inhibits plaque accumulation in the arteries
- Increases circulation
- Increases growth hormone production

- Builds muscle
- Enhances fat metabolism
- Increases sperm count
- Enhances immune function
- Vital for protein production
- Important for gut health
- Reduces pain from claudication (poor circulation)
- Helps wounds heal
- Decreases platelet stickiness

Natural sources of arginine are in beans, brewer's yeast, chocolate, dairy products, eggs, fish, legumes, meats, nuts, oatmeal, popcorn, raisins, seafood, seeds, sesame seeds, soy, sunflower seeds, whey, green peas, asparagus, broccoli, Swiss chard, corn, potatoes, onion, spinach, avocados, and whole grains.[46,47] For some people, supplementation may increase herpes simplex outbreaks (cold sores).

Dosage: 1,000–3,000 mg

Excitatory neurotransmitters increase the ability to send signals in the body and have an excitatory effect. The excitatory neurotransmitters include epinephrine, norepinephrine, PEA (phenylethylamine), histamine, aspartic acid, and glutamate. The interrelationship of these neurotransmitters and weight gain are now being researched.[48,49,50]

Epinephrine is an excitatory neurotransmitter that is also known as adrenaline. It regulates attentiveness and mental focus. It is made in the adrenal glands from norepinephrine. It is secreted in response to fear and anger.

Norepinephrine is synthesized from dopamine and is another excitatory neurotransmitter. It is important for focused attention and contributes to anxiety if levels are abnormal. Norepinephrine needs copper and vitamin C as cofactors to work in the body.

PEA is another one of the excitatory neurotransmitters. It is made from phenylalanine and promotes energy and elevates mood.

It inhibits the reuptake of dopamine and norepinephrine. Low levels of PEA are associated with depression. High levels are associated with schizophrenia. It may be also related to migraine headaches.

Histamine is also an excitatory neurotransmitter and has a pacemaker function in the brain. Aspartic acid is yet another excitatory neurotransmitter. It is made from glutamate.

Glutamate is the major excitatory neurotransmitter in the brain used by 70% of the excitatory synapses. Glutamate affects three different types of receptors in the body, including NMDA (N-methyl-D-aspartate) receptors, which play a role in controlling the body's ability to adapt to environmental and genetic influences. It is also involved in pain control and is concerned with sensory perception, memory, orientation in time and space, cognition, and motor skills. Any process that dramatically increases the activity of glutamate often causes the death of neurons. Glutamate is made from glutamine. Glutamine is a precursor for GABA and aids in decreasing food cravings and promoting weight loss. Glutamine is an amino acid that has numerous other functions in the body, which include:[51,52,53,54,55,56,57,58,59]

- Balancing blood sugar
- Maintaining a healthy gut
- Needed for the metabolism and maintenance of muscle
- Is a fueling source for the immune system
- Needed for DNA synthesis
- Promoting wound healing and tissue repair
- Neutralizing toxins
- Glutathione support
- Promotion of growth
- Increasing energy
- Improving mental alertness
- Promoting a healthy acid-alkaline balance in the body
- Helping the brain dispose of toxins such as ammonia
- Fighting cold and flu
- Elevating growth hormone levels
- Protecting the body from stress

Food sources of glutamine are beans, brewer's yeast, brown rice, dairy products, eggs, fish, legumes, meat, nuts, seafood, seeds, soy, whey, and whole grains.[60] If you have a sensitivity to MSG (monosodium glutamate), you should use glutamine with caution because it makes glutamate. MSG is an excitotoxin to the brain. The amount of MSG being added to prepared foods has doubled every decade since the 1940s.[61] It is added to most soups, chips, fast foods, frozen foods, ready-made diners, and canned goods. If you are taking medications for seizure disorders, only take glutamine under the direction of a physician.

Dosage: 500–3,000 mg

Glutamate is also available from alpha-ketoglutarate, which is a product of glucose metabolism. Glucose is a carbohydrate needed by the brain for functioning. In fact, 25% of the carbohydrates that go into the body are used by the brain for fueling. That is why it is very important for you to intake low glycemic index carbohydrates since they provide a better fueling source for the brain and the remainder of the body.

Dopamine is a unique neurotransmitter in the fact that it has both inhibitory and excitatory functions. Dopamine is made from tyrosine, and it makes epinephrine and norepinephrine in the body. It plays a role in the cardiovascular, renal (kidney), hormonal, and central nervous systems. Dopamine controls many processes in the body from movement to optimal weight maintenance to drug addiction. It more commonly functions as an excitatory neurotransmitter.

What causes neurotransmitter disorders? They occur when the current levels of neurotransmitters are unable to properly relay the electrical signal from one neuron to the next. Too high or too low levels of neurotransmitters can be a problem since they both can cause inappropriate signals. Low levels can occur due to prolonged stress, genetic predisposition, and a diet low in amino acids. Abnormal levels are associated with weight gain and obesity.

Neurotransmitters and their metabolites (breakdown products) can now be tested by urine testing (see Appendix). There is a significant variation that may occur with neurotransmitter levels. Consequently, there are observed ranges and optimal ranges. It is the goal of all practitioners to have their patients functioning in the optimal range. Therapeutic ranges have also been determined by some laboratories for those patients who are on targeted amino acid therapies to improve neurotransmitter function. Neurotransmitter testing is in its infancy. As research progresses in this field, new testing will become available to help people achieve optimal health. You may have many combinations of results depending on your original symptoms. For example, weight gain is frequently associated with low epinephrine and high norepinephrine levels. However, since the cause of weight gain is multifactorial, other symptoms such as insomnia, depression, anxiety, and abnormal stress levels also have to be considered. Abnormal neurotransmitter patterns that may also be commonly associated with these symptoms include:

- Insomnia:
  - High epinephrine
  - High norepinephrine
  - High GABA
  - High PEA
  - High glycine
  - Low serotonin
- Depression:
  - High glutamate
  - Low serotonin
  - Low norepinephrine
  - Low histamine
  - Low agmatine
- Anxiety:
  - High epinephrine
  - High GABA
  - High aspartic acid
  - High glycine
  - Low agmatine
- Abnormal stress levels:
  - High epinephrine
  - High norepinephrine
  - High or low serotonin
  - High histamine

There are many cofactors and precursors that are associated with normal neurotransmitter function. These include 5-HTP, tyroisine, phenylalanine, vitamins B6, B12, and folic acid, cystine, vitamin C, calcium citrate, selenium, mucuna, theanine, taurine, and rhodiola.

There are also hormonal effects that occur on neurotransmitters. The body is a chemical web, and just like the hormonal symphony that was discussed previously, there is an interplay between neurotransmitters and hormones. For example, from the previous chapter on stress hormones, it is apparent that they are affected by neurotransmitter function. Cortisol reduces anxiety and stress by decreasing the release of epinephrine and norepinephrine. It also increases the GABA receptors, thus providing a calming effect. DHEA enhances the neurotransmission of serotonin and norephinephrine. Consequently, it has both a calming and excitation affect on the body. Estrogen (estradiol) has an anti-dopamine effect. It also decreases MAO (monoamine oxidase), which is responsible for the inactivation of serotonin and dopamine. Progesterone increases GABA receptors and reduces neurotransmitter activity, thereby having a calming effect in women. Progesterone also increases MAO synthesis. Melatonin is made from serotonin under the regulation of norepeinephrine. Low levels of melatonin are associated with insomnia and reduced restfulness from sleep.

Drug companies have developed medications that are called reuptake inhibitors. Their purpose is to block the reuptake of neurotransmitters in the body so that their action lasts longer. For example, Lexapro™ prevents reuptake of serotonin. Others, such as Wellbutrin™, prevent the reuptake of norepinephrine. Still others, such as Effexor™, affect the reuptake of both serotonin and norepinephrine.

You may have imbalances of a single neurotransmitter or multiple neurotransmitters. Therapy can therefore be targeted to one or multiple abnormalities of neurotransmitter function. Treatment can include both nutritional support along with medications. As previously described, some nutrients cannot be used in conjunction with pharmaceuticals. Diets that are low in amino acids can limit neurotransmitter production. Therefore, a change in diet or amino acid supplementation can be an effective modality to treat neurotransmitter dysfunction.

The Science Behind Food Addictions 16

There are some food habits that are hard to break when you look at weight loss because they are physically addicting. Chocolate, cheese, and wheat are such substances, as is sugar.

Rather have chocolate than sex? The same part of the brain that appreciates chocolate is also responsible for libido.[1] Chocolate has opiate effects. It stimulates the release of chemicals within the brain's pleasure center that encourage you to be addicted. Chocolate stimulates the same part of your brain that morphine acts on. Chocolate is rich in a chemical called theobromine. This substance is a stimulant similar to caffeine. Chocolate also contains phenylethylamine, which is an amphetamine-like chemical.[2] Chocolate furthermore contains traces of substances similar to THC, which is the active ingredient in marijuana. Brain cells contain a chemical called anandamide, which is related to THC. Certain chemicals in chocolate delay the breakdown of anandamide in the brain so that the wonderful pleasant effects last longer than normal.[3]

Cheese and dairy products have a similar effect on your body as chocolate. Mild opiates are released during digestion of cheese and other dairy products.[4] Furthermore, milk contains a protein called casein. When casein breaks down during digestion, it releases a group of opiates called casomorphins. A cup of cow's milk contains six grams of casein. Skim milk has more. Cow's milk is high in casein and low in whey. Human breast milk is just the opposite. It is low in casein and high in whey protein. Cheese contains a lot more casein than milk. It also contains phenylethylamine, which is the same amphetamine-like chemical found in chocolate and sausage. A recent study found that men who avoid dairy products have a 30% reduction in the risk of prostate cancer.[5]

Of course, sugar is also addicting. It causes the release of opiates in the brain. In addition, sugar has an appetite-driving effect. Carbohydrate-rich foods boost serotonin, the neurotransmitter that helps regulate mood and sleep. Serotonin, as you have seen earlier, has a large influence on your eating behavior. If your food intake is low in tryptophan, it leads to low serotonin levels, which your brain senses as a state of starvation. Therefore, your appetite is stimulated. Serotonin levels decrease when dieting. This is why I never suggest putting a person on a diet. Studies have shown that you only gain weight, even if you have initially lost it. You want to be on a healthy eating program, which is a lifestyle change not a fad diet plan. Also, when you diet, your body's leptin system is impaired.[6] Your body goes into a "fight or flight response," and it burns no calories because it is storing them for later usage. There is only one way that your body stores food longer term and that is in fat cells. Lastly, wheat contains a protein called gluten. When gluten is metabolized, it is broken down into compounds that have a variety of mild opiate effects.

Other neurotransmitters are also affected by eating habits. PET scan studies show that many overweight people have fewer brain receptors for dopamine (DRD2) compared to people who are not overweight. Therefore, this brain-rewarding chemical has fewer receptor sites to help the person feel good. Consequently, you may overeat to get the pleasurable stimulation that you may lack.[7]

An excellent book on food addictions is *Breaking the Food Seduction* by Neal Barnard.[8]

Nutrients That Aid in Weight Loss 17

As you have already seen from the previous chapters in this book, nutrients are very important to help the body function optimally. Consequently, having the right amount of vitamins, minerals, amino acids, fatty acids, and other nutrients is a key element in obtaining and maintaining weight loss. Nutrients are needed to make your sex hormones and also to help you deal with stress. Vitamins, minerals, and amino acids are also required to make thyroid hormones. Insulin resistance, inflammation, and free radical production can be treated with neutraceuticals. Likewise, many nutrients are used to help your body detoxify and to restore bowel health. Furthermore, your body requires zinc, magnesium, and vitamins for the conversion of fatty acids into proteins. Supplements can even help you sleep better and can fight yeast-related health problems. The chemical pathways in your system called neurotransmitters require many cofactors and precursors that are nutritional. Therefore, nutrients are a key element in your fight to lose weight and keep it off.

Every year over 75% of your body is replaced and reconstructed from the nutrients you eat and take, even the DNA of your genes. The quality of these vitamins and nutrients determines the quality of your cells, how well they function, prevent disease, and how easy it is for you to lose weight.

Vitamin supplements are divided into four quality categories.[1]

Pharmaceutical grade. This grade meets the highest regulatory requirements for purity, dissolution, and absorption. There is outside verification as to the quality.

Medical grade. This grade is a high-grade product. Prenatal vitamins usually fit into this category.

Cosmetic, nutritional grade. Supplements of this grade are often not tested for purity, dissolution, or absorption and may not have a high concentration of the active ingredient they are labeled as.

Feed or agricultural grade. Supplements of this grade are used for veterinary purposes. Do not take supplements of this grade.

The chemical structures of minerals are not elemental forms, and this also makes a difference in the nutrients that you are taking. For example, a 1,200 mg tablet of calcium gluconate is only 9% elemental. This means that it only contains 108 mg of calcium. You would therefore need to take 11 capsules or tablets a day to get the recommended amount.[2] In addition, natural or synthetic forms also make a difference with vitamins such as vitamin E. Natural vitamin E is better absorbed and more active than synthetic.[3]

Your herbal supplements should have an adulteration screen done to see if there are any toxic metals present, such as arsenic, lead, mercury, or cadmium. They should also be screened for contaminants such as other pharmaceuticals and be analyzed for pesticides, fungicides, insecticides, and other toxic ingredients.[4]

Many forms of nutrients are hardly bioavailable, and they pass through your gut without being absorbed. For example, magnesium oxide is only one-tenth as bioavailable as magnesium aspartate.[5] However, manufacturers will frequently use the oxide form because the aspartate form is more expensive and takes up a lot of room in the capsule.

The dosages discussed throughout this book are for adults and are daily amounts. All dosages are in milligrams (mg) unless otherwise stated. If milligrams are not used, the units of dosage are spelled out to avoid confusion. One thousand micrograms equal one mg, and 1,000 mg equal one gram.

Almost 75% of your health and life expectancy is based on lifestyle, environment, and nutrition.[6] So is your ability to lose weight and to keep it off. Medications, vitamin interaction, soil depletion, need for more antioxidants, stress, age, lifestyle, and genetics all play a role in determining which nutrients are right for you. The recommended daily allowances (RDAs) and the reference daily intakes (RDIs) are designed to prevent disease. They are not designed for optimal health. The RDAs and RDIs, furthermore, do not take into account that the amount of vitamins, minerals, and other nutrients you need are not the same as what someone else needs.

Here are some examples of how medications may deplete your body of specific vitamins and minerals. Vitamins can also increase or decrease the absorption of your medications.[7]

- Long-term use of antacids (prescription or over-the-counter) can lead to decreased folic acid absorption.
- Regular use of aspirin decreases folate levels.
- Birth control pills and other forms of estrogen replacement deplete your body of B vitamins.
- Too much vitamin B6 can decrease the effectiveness of levadopa.
- Disopyramide (Norpace) and quinidine sulfate can cause magnesium deficiency.
- Colchicine reduces the absorption of beta-carotene and also probably magnesium, potassium, and vitamin B12.
- Methotrexate decreases beta-carotene, folic acid, and vitamin B12.
- Estrogen replacement increases calcium absorption.

- Seizure medications (anticonvulsants) can deplete your body of carnitine.
- H2 blockers (used to treat reflux), such as cimetidine, decrease vitamin D activity.
- HMG-CoA reductase inhibitors used to lower cholesterol (statin drugs) stop your body from making coenzyme Q-10.
- Medications to lower blood sugar, such as glyburide (Diabeta), acetohexamide (Dymelor), and tolazamide (Tolinase), all can lead to coenzyme Q-10 deficiency.
- Digoxin can increase the rate of calcium excretion from your body.
- Fiber can decrease the absorption of digoxin.
- Diuretics (water pills) increase the loss of magnesium, potassium, sodium, and zinc.
- Calcium can decrease the absorption of beta blockers.
- Potassium-sparing diuretics deplete your body of folic acid, calcium, and zinc.

If you are on any of the above medications, it is important that your doctor or other healthcare professional aids you in replacing the nutrients depleted or makes sure that your vitamins and your medications do not interact. This will keep you stay healthier and increase your ability to lose weight.

Second, even the foods you eat can affect the medication you are taking. For example, be aware that grapefruit may increase the risk of side effects of the following medications:[8]

- Calcium-channel blockers (e.g., nifedipine, amlodipine, verapamil, felodipine) if taken with grapefruit can decrease blood pressure, cause flushing, headache, and increased heart rate.
- Grapefruit increases the levels of quinidine.
- Grapefruit can cause irregular heart rhythms if you are taking terfenadine.

- If you are taking a sedative (benzodiazepines, e.g., alprazolam, diazepam, midazolam, triazolam), grapefruit can increase levels of the medication.
- Grapefruit increases estrogen levels for both men and women.
- If you are taking cyclosporine, grapefruit increases the levels and can cause kidney and liver toxicity.
- Grapefruit increases the level of caffeine in your body and can cause nervousness and insomnia.
- If you are taking a macrolide antibiotic, such as clarithromycin, grapefruit will decrease its absorption.
- If you are taking fexofenadine (Allegra), grapefruit decreases the absorption of the medication.
- If you are taking statin drugs (HMG-CoA reductase inhibitors), grapefruit may increase the medication level.
- Grapefruit increases the levels of warfarin.
- Grapefruit delays the absorption of Viagra.
- Grapefruit and naprosyn taken together may cause hives.
- If you are taking carbamazepine (Tegretol), grapefruit can increase levels, which may lead to nausea, tremors, drowsiness, dizziness, or agitation.
- If you are taking amiodarone, grapefruit may elevate blood levels, and you may have nausea, drowsiness, tremors, or agitation.

Third, vitamins and minerals and other nutrients can also interact with each other. They do not exist in a vacuum. The nutrients have relationships and interrelationships with other nutrients. If interactions occur, they can interfere with your ability to lose weight effectively. The following are examples of how vitamins and minerals interact:[9,10,11,12]

- You have to have enough vitamin C in your body to use selenium effectively.
- Vitamin C can enhance the availability of vitamin A.

- Zinc in excess can decrease calcium absorption.
- Vitamin D increases the absorption of calcium and magnesium.
- Vitamin D helps your body use zinc effectively.
- Too much copper can decrease the uptake of manganese in your system.
- Vitamin A deficiency can decrease iron utilization.
- Too much iron can lower your manganese and copper levels.
- Too much riboflavin (vitamin B2) can cause magnesium deficiency.
- Vitamin B6 can cause a decrease in copper absorption.
- Vitamin A absorption may be lower if vitamin E levels are not adequate.
- Vitamin B6 deficiency can lead to a decreased use of selenium.
- Adequate phosphorus intake is needed to maintain vitamin D.

Fourth, in today's world you cannot get all the nutrients you need from food because of the following reasons:

- The soil is deplete of many minerals, such as zinc and magnesium. Selenium may be deplete or in overabundance in the ground depending on where you live. If the soil the fruits and vegetables are grown in is not rich in nutrients, then the food you eat will not contain an adequate supply of minerals.
- Fruits and vegetables begin to lose their nutritional value immediately after being picked. Cold storage causes destruction of nutrients. Stored grapes lose up to 30% of their B vitamins. Tangerines stored for 8 weeks can lose almost half of their vitamin C. Asparagus stored for one week loses up to 90% of its vitamin C. [13,14]
- The nutrients in your food may not be in a form that is bioavailable. In other words, it will not be easily absorbed into your body. Orange juice is an example: 40% of the vitamin C in orange juice is biologically inactive.

- Processing (blanching, sterilizing, canning, and freezing) decreases the nutritional value of the food you eat.
- The longer you cook fruits and vegetables, the less nutrition remains. Therefore, eat them raw or steamed lightly.
- The milling of grains removes 26 essential nutrients and much of the fiber.[15]

For more information concerning this subject, read *The New Nutrition* by Michael Colgan, Ph.D., *Dr. Art Ulene's Complete Guide to Vitamins, Minerals, and Herbs* by Art Ulene, M.D., or *The Real Vitamin and Mineral Book* by Shari Lieberman, Ph.D. It is important that when you begin a healthy eating program to lose weight that you also take a good multivitamin and a pharmaceutical grade fish oil (EPA/DHA) to provide an adequate amount of vitamins, minerals, and other nutrients to help the body burn calories and decrease inflammation.

Diet and nutritional states also play a major role in influencing how your genes express themselves, which also affects your ability to lose weight and decreases your risk of developing diseases such as diabetes. As Dr. Leo Galland points out "it depends as much upon the milieu in which a gene functions as it does upon the DNA sequence of the genome."[16] In other words, even if you have inherited a gene for a particular disease such as Alzheimer=s disease, whether you go on to have the disease is very much dependent on your environment, the food you eat, the toxins you are around, your stress level, and the nutrients you take in. Dr. Roger Williams discusses this situation in his book *Biochemical Individuality: The Basis for the Genotropic Concept*. He states, "Nutrition applied with due concern for individual genetic variations, which may be large, offers the solution to many baffling health problems." Your body is a lot like a car. If you put in good fuel (food and nutrients), it will run well, need little repair, and last a long time. If you put low octane fuel in your premium car (your body), your body will not run well; it will develop disease, and you will not live as long. You will also not lose weight as effectively if you are not fueling your body with the best nutrients available.

Scientific studies have shown that two nutrients are effective to aid with weight loss. They are CLA (conjugated linoleic acid) and L-carnitine.

CLA is a naturally occurring fatty acid. It not only aids in weight loss, but it also has been found to lower cholesterol, fight cancer, build the immune system, and improve insulin sensitivity. It is also an antioxidant.[17,18,19,20,21,22,23,24] The recommended dosage of CLA for weight loss is 3,000 to 4,000 mg a day.

L-carnitine is an amino acid. It is made from lysine and methionine in your liver, kidneys, and brain. Your body also uses niacin, vitamin B6, iron, and vitamin C to synthesize L-carnitine. This amino acid has many other functions in the body besides helping to promote weight loss.

Functions of L-carnitine:[25,26,27,28,29,30]

- Needed for the transport of long-chain fatty acids into the cells
- Helps convert stored body fat into energy
- Energizes the heart
- Reduces triglycerides
- Lowers cholesterol
- Raises HDL (good cholesterol)
- May slow the progression of Alzheimer's disease
- Prevents DNA degeneration
- Promotes DNA repair from nutraitons that occur from free radical production
- Reduces the buildup of acids and metabolic waste
- Increases oxygen availability and respiratory efficiency
- Can be converted to acetyl choline in the body
- Improves mental focus and energy
- Enhances energy and long-term memory

There are many things that can cause your body to have low levels of L-carnitine. If you are deficient in vitamins C, B6, and B12, folic acid, iron, lysine or SAMe, you may be deplete in this important nutrient. If you are taking valproic acid, pivampicillin, sulfadiazine, or pyrimethamine, you may have less L-carnitine than your body needs to function optimally. Also, if you are a vegetarian, you may have low L-carnitine levels since the main dietary source of L-carnitine is found in red meat.[31] As previously discussed, nutrients in the body do not function by themselves. They interact with each other. Phosphatidylserine, B vitamins, alpha lipoic acid, phosphatidyl choline, and EPA/DHA (fish oil) all help L-carnitine work more effectively. The dosage for weight loss for L-carnitine supplementation is 3,000 to 4,000 mg a day. You should consult your doctor before you start taking L-carnitine if you have kidney or liver disease. Acetyl-L-carnitine is the form of L-carnitine that is effective in helping maintain cognition.

Another nutrient that may be helpful to lose weight and help keep it off is ningxia wolfberry. The Lycium barbarum L. form is the most effective. Wolfberry is a fruit that is low on the glycemic index. It is high in fiber and protein and contains many nutrients. It has 67 times the nutritional value of B1 as brown rice, two times the amount of niacin as baker's yeast, and three times the value of vitamin C as raw oranges.[32] Ningxia wolfberry contains many other nutrients, such as lutein, zeaxanthin, potassium, magnesium, zinc, arginine, ellagic acid, chromium, and calcium. In fact, ningxia wolfberry contains more calcium than cottage cheese.[33] Studies done in Australia revealed that calcium intake at a higher dose is associated with lower body mass index (BMI) and waist size.[34] However, clinical trials have shown that dairy sources of calcium are not as effective for weight loss.[35] Studies conducted on vegetable sources of calcium, however, revealed the opposite. Those who ingested higher levels of calcium-rich foods from vegetables tended toward a lower BMI.[36] Therefore, fruit sources of calcium, such as wolfberry, are ideally suited to aid in the weight-loss battle. Furthermore, ningzia wolfberry also helps satisfy hunger cravings.[37] For availability of this fruit, see the Appendix.

Weight loss of 20 pounds or more may precipitate a gallstone attack. Nutrients that aid the function of the gallbladder and liver are helpful in preventing gallstones. Alpha lipoic acid, dandelion, milk thistle (silymarin), and other nutrients have been found to be helpful. In our practice, we use LV-GB made by Designs for Health (see Appendix for availability).

CONCLUSION

By now, I am sure it is obvious to you that no one single eating program or weight loss method works for everyone. It takes only eating an extra 100 calories a day for you to gain five pounds a year. Why not just count calories then, if it is that simple? Studies done by nutritionists have shown that it is hard for even them to know how many calories that you have consumed in a day. So how can you be expected to be able to count calories when experts in the field are not able to count them accurately?

There are many reasons why you have an appetite. It is regulated by your brain-gut connection, which is part of the autonomic nervous system. Your messenger cells, neurotransmitters, are also important. Other messenger cells called cytokines, which are part of your immune system, also govern your hunger needs. Your appetite is also regulated by your metabolic hormones such as insulin, thyroid, and your sex hormones. They all work together to assist your body as to when and how much to eat. If your body is not functioning optimally, then your system gets mixed messages. You will, therefore, not know when to eat or the amount to eat to keep your weight at an optimal level. Consequently, willpower has little to do with whether you can lose weight and keep it off.

In the final analysis, medications and surgery for weight loss have limited effect because of the interactions between your body's systems.[2,3] Changing any one component has little effect on the long-term issues of weight gain. If you use appetite suppressants or weight-loss programs that are not healthy, you not only may gain the weight back when they are stopped but will also frequently add an additional ten pounds. Successful weight management is done only through optimizing hormonal function, including insulin, thyroid, stress hormones, and sex hormones. Two newly discovered hormones, which have not been discussed previously in this book, that affect weight are grehliln and PYY. Grehliln is produced in the stomach and is responsible for making you feel hungry. PYY is secreted also by the stomach, and this hormone makes you feel full. When these hormones are out of balance, it is hard for you to determine when to eat and when to stop dining. Research is now being conducted on these hormones. Inflammation, toxic buildup, and neurotransmitter dysfunction also contribute to weight gain. Even how well you sleep affects your weight. The focus on the treatment of weight loss should not be on the "disease" itself, but on optimizing functional systems in the body that are unique to you.

Sugar is one of the most addicting substances on earth. It comes in many forms, sucrose, honey, glucose, maltose, dextrose, fructose, corn syrup, lactose, and even white grape juice. High fructose corn syrup is one of the most commonly used sweeteners in the United States. It accounts for more than 40% of the total sweeteners consumed.[4] High fructose corn syrup, when processed, is absorbed into the body at a faster rate than regular sugar (glucose plus fructose) because it does not need help in being absorbed whereas glucose requires insulin to help it enter your cells. A high intake of high fructose corn syrup can also lead to elevated cholesterol and triglyceride levels. Furthermore, high fructose corn syrup does not increase leptin, which, if elevated, would decrease your appetite. Fructose is the sugar that is contained in fruit, but the metabolization effects of fructose in fruit are different because of the high fiber content of fruit. An excellent article on this subject by Dr. Mark Hyman appeared in *Alternative Therapies* recently.[5] The use of artificial sweeteners, such as aspartame, may lead to increased food intake.[6,7]

It does matter what time of day you eat and how frequently you dine. Your body makes insulin around 10:00 in the morning and around 4:00 in the afternoon. It is important to eat before 10:00 A.M. so that insulin will work more effectively in your body. Studies have shown that people who skip breakfast eat more food and more easily develop insulin resistance.[8] Eating five to six small meals a day improves weight loss and decreases the number of calories eaten.[9,10]

Low glycemic index meals have been shown to promote weight loss more than low-fat meals. In many low-fat foods, the fat has been taken out, and sugar has been added. Medical studies have revealed that low-fat programs slow your metabolism more than low glycemic index meals.[11] The amount of fiber in your diet also affects your ability to lose weight and to keep it off. Fiber slows down the process of digestion, which improves satiety, increases fat burning, and reduces the amount of insulin that your body produces. In all of these ways, high-fiber meals help you lose weight. Clinical trials have shown that high-fiber diets are associated with weight loss and lower insulin levels.[12]

Two new fibers being studied are of interest. They are konjac root and rye.[13] Konjac, Amorphophallus konjac K Koch, is an Asian root. It is very effective in lowering cholesterol and slows the rate of absorption of meals. It is being studied at the University of Toronto.[14] Rye fiber has been shown in studies to lower blood sugar and insulin more than other fibers.[15]

It is important, while you look at weight loss and how to keep it off, not to "beat yourself up." If you "fall off the wagon" and eat something that is high in caloric value, just get right back on the wagon. Everyone eats things that are not healthy. The goal is to minimize the number of times you eat these kinds of foods. After you are at your goal weight, the idea is that you have achieved a lifestyle change, not that you have been on a diet and now you are not on one. What I do myself, and suggest to my patients, is to take one night a week and eat the dessert or other high-caloric food that you crave after you have achieved your goal weight. It is much easier to keep the weight off if you know that once a week you can eat any food you want. This does include alcohol. Alcohol is a sugar and is considered a "sweet."

In short, *Demystifying Weight Loss*, has introduced you to a new way of looking at medicine. It is a functional approach. This book has looked at antecedents to weight gain, which are congenital and developmental issues, such as exposure to toxins, nutrition, psychological issues, and the effects of antibiotics on the microbial ecology of the gut. Understanding the precipitating events may aid in looking at the triggers and mediators that maintain your weight gain. This book has also examined these triggers, such as stress, which initiate the problem of weight gain. Mediators are anything that produces symptoms that may damage tissues of the body, as well as the types of behaviors associated with weight gain. Mediators include items such as hormonal and neurotransmitter dysfunction, free radical production and inflammation, and abnormal gut flora secondary to yeast and overuse of antibiotics. Weight gain and obesity are very complex medical disorders that require a multifaceted approach. Consequently, it is important to individualize and customize your program. One size does not fit all. It is helpful to seek the aid of a practitioner who is fellowship trained in anti-aging and functional medicine (see Appendix for availability).

APPENDIX

All lab testing referenced in this book is available through:

Genova Diagnostic Laboratory
63 Zillicoa St.
Asheville, NC 28801-1074
1-800-522-4762
www.gsdl.com

ImmunoScience, Inc.
325 S 3rd St., #1-107
Las Vegas, NV 89101
1-925-460-8111
www.immunoscience.com

Age Diagnostic Laboratories
1341 W Fullerton Ave., Suite 123
Chicago, IL 60614
1-773-528-8500
www.adltests.com

NeuroScience
373 280th St.
Osceola, WI 54020
1-715-755-3995
www.neurorelief.com

ZRT Laboratory
1815 NW 169th Pl., Suite 5050
Beaverton, OR 97006
1-503-466-2445
www.zrtlab.com

Supplements from the following companies are only available through your healthcare professional or local compounding pharmacy.

Metagenics
P.O. Box 1729
Gig Harbor, WA 98335
1-800-843-9660
www.metagenics.com

Ortho Molecular Products
3017 Business Park Drive
P.O. Box 1060
Stevens Point, WI 54481
1-800-332-2351

Designs For Health
2 North Road
East Windsor, CT 06088
1-800-847-8302
www.DesignsForHealth.com

Billie Sahley, Ph.D.
Pain & Stress Center
5282 Medical Drive, Suite 160
San Antonio, TX 78229
1-800-669-2256
www.painstresscenter.com

For a compounding pharmacy near you, contact:

Professional Compounding Centers of America
9901 South Wilcrest Dr.
Houston, TX 77099
1-800-331-2498
www.pccarx.com

REFERENCES

Introduction

1. Centers for Disease Control and Prevention, National Center on Vital Statistics, 2003, table 68.
2. Bloch, A., "Obesity: the challenge for the healthcare professional," *Issues and Choices in Clinical Nutrition Practice*. Philadelphia: Lippincott Williams & Wilkins, 2007, p. 319.
3. Serdula, M., et al., "Do obese children become obese adults? A review of the literature," *Pre Med* 1993; 22: 167–77.
4. Ibid., p. 167–77.
5. Ibid., Bloch, p. 319.
6. Mokdad, A., et al., "Actual causes of death in the United States, 2000," *JAMA* 2004; 291: 1238–45.
7. Flegal, K., et al., "Excess deaths associated with underweight, overweight, and obesity," *JAMA* 2005; 293: 1861–67.
8. Wechsler, H., HHS efforts to combat the obesity epidemic among children and adolescents. Testimony before the Subcommittee on Oversight ad Investigations, Committee on Energy and Commerce, U.S. House of Representatives. Available at: http://www.hhs.govb/asl/testify/t040616.html.

   and Ibid., Bloch, p. 320.
9. Strum, R., "The effects of obesity, smoking, and drinking on medical problems and costs," *Health Affairs* 2002; 21: 235–53.

Chapter 1: Allergies and Weight Loss

1. Gaby, A., "The role of hidden food allergy in chronic disease," *Alt Med Rev* 1998; 3(2): 90–100.
2. Appleton, N., *Stopping Inflammation: Relieving the Cause of Degenerative Diseases.* Garden City Park, NY: Square One Publishers, 2005.

3. Ibid., p. 20.

4. Edwards, T., et al., "Failure to thrive," *Clinical and Environmental Allergy*, 1995; 25: 16–19.

5. Ibid., Appleton, p. 26.

6. Ibid., Appleton, p. 49.

7. Rothenberg, M., et al., "A pathological function for exotoxin and eosinophils in eosinophilic gastrointestinal inflammation," *Nature Immunology* 2001; 2: 353–60.

8. Marshall, P., et al., "Effects of seasonal allergic rhinitis on fatigue levels and mood," *Psychosm Med* 2002 64(4): 684–91.

Chapter 2: Stress Hormones and Weight Loss

1. Goldman, B., *Brain Fitness*. New York: Doubleday, 1999, p. 140.

2. Benson, H., *The Relaxation Response*. New York: Quill Publishers, 2001.

3. Ahlgrimm, M., *The HRT Solution*. 1999; New York: Avery Publishing, p. 28.

4. Barbieri, R., et al., "Cotinine and nicotine inhibit human fetal adrenal 11, beta-hydroxylase," *Jour Clin Endocrinol Metab* 1989; 69: 1221–24.

5. Ibid., p. 1221–24.

6. Yeh, J., et al., "Nicotine and cotinine inhibit rat testes androgen biosynthesis in vitro," *Jour Steroid Biochem* 1989; 33(4A): 627–30.

7. Lieberman, S., *The Real Vitamin and Mineral Book*. New York: Avery Publishing, 1997; p. 220.

8. Barrett-Conner, E., et al., "A prospective study of dehydroepiandrosterone sulfate, mortality and cardiovascular disease," *NEJM* 1986; 37(9); 1035.

9. Brownstein, D., *Overcoming Thyroid Disorders*. West Bloomfield MI: Medical Alternatives Press, 2002, p. 140.

10. Gordon, G., et al., "Reduction of atherosclerosis by administration of dehydroepiandrosterone. A study of the hypercholesterolemic New Zealand white rabbit and aortic internal injury," *Jour Clin Invest* 1988; 82: 712.

11. Heller, L., *The Essentials of Herbal Care Part II*. San Clemente, CA: Metagenics, Inc., 2000; p. 1144.

12. Ibid., p. 1145.

13. Vliet, E., *Women, Weight and Hormones*. New York: M. Evans & Company, 2001; p. 129.

14. Ibid., Heller, p. 1145.

15. Ibid., Vliet, p. 140.

16. Ibid., Heller, p. 1144.

17. Bland, J., "Introduction to neuroendocrine disorders," *Functional Medicine Approaches to Endocrine Disturbances of Aging,* Gig Harbor, Washington: The Functional Medicine Institute, 2001; p. 121.

18. Ibid., Vliet, p. 129.

19. Wilson, J., *Adrenal Fatigue.* Petaluma, CA: Smart Publications, 2001; p. [MISSING PG. #]

20. Wilson, J., "Metabolic syndrome and adrenal fatigue: balancing the difficult patient," *BHRT for Female Patients Symposium*, Houston, Texas, August 24–26, 2006; p. 36.

21. Ibid., p. 37–8, 43–4, 46–8.

22. Ibid., p. 45–6.

23. Ibid., p. 49.

24. Ibid., Vliet, p. 140.

25. Bjomtop, P., et al., "Consolatory eating is not a myth. Stress-induced cortisol levels result in leptin-resistant obesity," *Lakartidningen* 2001; 98(48): 5458–61.

26. Stewart, P., et al., "Growth hormone, insulin-like growth factor-1 and the cortisol-cortisone shuttle," *Hormone Research* 2001; 56: 1–6.

27. Epel, E., et al., "Can stress shape your body? Consistently greater stress-induced cortisol secretion among women with abdominal fat," *Psychosomatic Med* 2000; (62): 623–32.

28. Goldman, R., *Brain Fitness*. New York: Doubleday, 1999; p. 165.

29. Fulder, S., et al., "Ginseng and the hypothalamic pituitary control of stress," *Amer Jour Chinese Med* IX (2): 112–18.

30. Kelly, G., et al., "Nutritional and botanical interventions to assist with the adaption to stress," *Altern Med Rev* 1999; 4(4): 249–65.

31. Rege, N., et al., "Adaptogenic properties of six Rasuyana herbs used in ayurvedic medicine," *Phytotherapy Res* 1999; 13: 275–92.

32. Grandi, A., et al., "A comparative pharmacological investigation of ashwagandha and ginseng," *Jour Ethnopharmacol* 1994; 44: 131–35.

33. Darbinyan, VB., et al., "Rhodiola rosea in stress induced fatigue—a double-blind crossover study of a standardized extract SHR-J with a repeated low dose regimen on the mental performance of healthy physicians during night duty," *Phytomed* 2000; 7(5): 365–71.

34. Zhu, U., et al., "The scientific rediscovery of an ancient Chinese herbal medicine: Cordyceps sinensis," *Jour Alt Complem Med* 1998; 4(3): 289–03.

35. Tully, D., et al., "Modulation of steroid receptor-mediated gene expression by vitamin B6," *FASEB Jour* 1994; 8: 343–49.

36. Crayhon, R., "Aging well in the 21st century," *Seminar* 2002; p. 24.

37. Bland, J., "Normalizing HPA function," *Nutritional Endocrinology: Breakthrough Approaches for Improving Adrenal and Thyroid Function*. Gig Harbor, WA: The Functional Medicine Institute, 2002; p. 61–6.

Chapter 3: Female Hormones and Weight Loss

1. Laux, M., *Natural Woman, Natural Menopause*. New York: HarperCollins, 1997, p. 99.

2. Murray, M., *The Healing Power of Herbs*. California: Prima Publications, 1995, p. 375.

3. Ahene, S., et al., "Polycystic ovary syndrome," *Nurs Stand* 2004; 18(26): 40–4.

4. Atimo, W., et al., "Familial associations in women with polycystic ovary syndrome," *Fert Steril* 2003; 80(1): 143–45.

5. Gonzalez, C., et al., "Polycystic ovaries in childhood: a common finding in daughters of PCOS patients. A pilot study," *Hum Repro* 2002; 17(3): 771–76.

6. Strauss, J., et al., "Some new thoughts on the pathophysiology and genetics of polycystic ovary syndrome," *Ann NY Aci Sci* 2003; 997: 42–8.

7. Carey, A., et al., "Evidence for a single gene effect causing polycystic ovaries and male pattern baldness," *Clin Endocrinol* 38(6): 653–58.

8. Urbanek, M., et al., "Thirty-seven candidate genes for PCOS: Strongest evidence of linkage is follistatin," *Proc Nat Acd Aci* 1999; 38(6): 653–58.

9. Marantides, D., et al., "Management of polycystic ovary syndrome," *Nurse Pract* 1997; 22(12): 34–8, 40–1.

10. Tsilchorozidou, T., et al., "Altered cortisol metabolism in polycystic ovary syndrome: insulin enhances 5 alpha-reduction but not the elevated adrenal steroid production rates," *Jour Clin Endocrino Metab* 2003; 88(12): 5907–13.

11. Barnea, E., et al., "Stress-related reproductive failure," *Jour IVF Embryo Transfer* 1991; 8: 15–23.

12. Pelusi, B., et al., "Type 2 diabetes and the polycystic ovary syndrome," *Minerva Ginecol* 2004; 56(1): 41–51.

13. Gonzalez, C., et al., "Polycystic ovarian disease: clinical and biochemical expression," *Ginecol Obstet Mex* 2003; 71: 253–58.

14. Legro, R., et al., "Prevalence and predictors of risk for Type 2 diabetes mellitus and impaired glucose tolerance in polycystic ovary syndrome: a

prospective, controlled study in 254 affected women," *Jour Clin Endocrinol Metabol* 1999; 84(1): 165–69.

15. De Leo, V., et al., "Polycystic ovary syndrome and type 2 diabetes mellitus," *Minera Ginecol* 2004; 56(1): 53–62.

16. Solomon, C., et al., "Long or irregular menstrual cycle as a marker for the risk of type 2 diabetes mellitus," *JAMA* 2001; 286(19): 2421–26.

17. Robinson, S., et al., "Postprandial thermogenesis is reduced in polycystic ovary syndrome and is associated with increased insulin resistance," *Clin Endocrinol* (Oxf) 1992; 36(6): 537–43.

18. Falola, E., et al., "Body composition, fat distribution and metabolic characteristics in lean and obese women with polycystic ovary syndrome," *Jour Endocrinol Invest* 2004; 27(5): 424–29.

19. Gambineria, A., et al., "Obesity and the polycystic ovary syndrome," *Int Jour Obes Relat Metab Disord* 2002; 26(7): 883–96.

20. Smith, P., *Vitamins: Hype or Hope*. Traverse City, Michigan: Healthy Living Books, 2004, p. 210–11.

21. Harris, C, and Cheung, T., *The PCOS Protection Plan*. Carlsbad, CA: Hay House Inc. 2006.

22. Smith, P., *HRT: The Answers*. Traverse City, Michigan: Healthy Living Books, 2003.

23. Sacks, F., et. al., "Sex hormones, lipoproteins, and vascular reactivity," *Curr Opin Lipodol* 1995; 6(3): 161–66.

24. Vliet, E., *Women Weight and Hormones*. New York: M. Evans & Company, 2001; p. 45.

25. Colacurci, N., et al., "Effects of hormone replacement therapy on glucose metabolism," *Panminerva Med* 1998; 40(1): 18–21.

26. Anderson, B., et al., "Estrogen replacement therapy decreases hyperandrogenicity and improves glucose homeostasis: Plasma lipids in postmenopausal women with NIDDM," *Jour Clin Endocrin* 1997; 82(2): 638–43.

27. Ibid., Vliet, p. 45.

28. Ibid., Vliet, p. 145.

29. Lee, J., *What Your Doctor May Not Tell You About Premenopause*. New York: Warner Books, 1999, p. 4.

30. Bland, J., "Introduction to neuroendocrine disorders," *Functional Medicine Approaches to Endocrine Disturbances of Aging*. Gig Harbor, Washington: The Functional Medicine Institute, 2001; p. 65.

31. Ibid., Bland, p. 121.

32. Aldercreatz, J., et al., "Western diet and western diseases: some hormonal and biochemical mechanisms and associations," *Scand Jour Clin Lab Invest* 1990; 50 (Suppl 201).

33. Collins, J., *What's Your Menopause Type*. Roseville, CA: Prima Health, 2000; p. 285.

34. Ibid., Vliet, p. 81.

35. Ibid., Vliet, p. 81.

36. Ibid., Vliet, p. 217.

37. Ibid., Vliet, p. 88.

38. Ibid., Vliet, p. 203.

39. Ibid., Bland, p. 121.

40. Ibid., Vliet, p. 69.

41. Lemon, H., et al., "Estriol prevention of mammary carcinoma induced by 7, 12–dimethylbenzanthracene and procarbazine," *Cancer Res* 1975; 35: 1341–352.

42. Lemon, H., et al., "Reduced estriol excretion in patients with breast cancer prior to endocrine therapy," *JAMA* 1966; 196(13): 1129–36.

43. Follingstad, A., "Estriol, the forgotten estrogen?" *JAMA* 1978; 239(1): 29–30.

44. Lemon, H., et al., "Pathophysiologic considerations in the treatment of menopausal symptoms with estrogens: the role of estriol in the prevention of mammary carcinoma," *ACTA Endocrinol* 1980; 233 (Suppl): 17–27.

45. Ibid., Laux, p. 79.

46. Ibid., Vliet, p. 81.

47. Ibid., Vliet, p. 218.

48. Pansini, F., et al., "Control of carbohydrate metabolism in menopausal women receiving transdermal estrogen therapy," *Ann NY Acad Sci* 1990; 592: 460–62.

49. Ibid., Vliet, p. 224.

50. Sinatra, S., *Heart Sense for Women*. Washington D.C.: LifeLine Press, 2000, p. 210.

51. The Postmenopausal Estrogen/Progestin Interventions (PEPI) trial: National Heart, Lung, and Blood Institute, Nov. 17, 1994; 1–4.

52. Bradlow, H., et al., "Effects of pesticides on the ratio of 16-alpha: 2-hydroxyestrone: a biologic marker of breast cancer risk," *Environ Health Prospect* 1995; 103(Suppl 17): 147–50.

53. Ibid., Bradlow, p. 147–50.

54. Bradlow, H., et al., "2-hydroxyestrone the 'good' estrogen," *Jour Endocrinol* 1996; 150 (Suppl): S259–S265.

55. Fishman, J., et al., "The role of estrogen in mammary carcinogenesis," *Ann NY Acad Sci* 1995; 768: 91–100.

56. Michnovicz, J., et al., "Introduction of estradiol metabolism by dietary indole-3-carbinol in humans," *Jour Nat Canc Inst* 1990; 82: 947–49.

57. Fishman, J., et al., "Biological properties of 16-alpha hydroxyl estrone: implications in estrogen physiology and pathophysiology," *Jour Clin Endocrinol Metabol* 1980; 51: 611–15.

58. Zhu, B., et al., "Is 2-methoxyestradiol an endogenous estrogen metabolite that inhibits mammary carcinogenesis?" *Cancer Res* 1998; 58: 2269–77.

59. Martucci, C., et al., "P450 enzymes of estrogen metabolism," *Pharmacol Ther* 1993; 57: 237–57.

60. Ursin, G., et al., "Urinary 2-hydroxy estrone/16 alpha hydroxyl estrone ratio: risk of breast cancer in postmenopausal women," *Jour Nat Canc Inst* 1999; 91: 1067–72.

61. Ibid., Bland, p. 91.

62. Meilahn, D., "Do urinary oestrogen metabolites predict breast cancer?" *Guersey III Cohort Follow-up* 1998; 78(9): 1250–55.

63. Ibid., Fishman, p. 611–615.

64. Fishman, J., et al., "Increased estrogen 16-alpha hydroxylase activity in women with breast and endometrial cancer," *Jour Steroid Biochem* 1984; 20: 1077–81.

65. Telang, N., et al., "Induction by estrogen metabolite 16-alpha hydroxyl estrone of genotoxic damage and aberrant proliferation in mouse mammory epithelial cells," *Jour Nat Cancer Inst* 1992; 84(8): 634–38.

66. Arnot, B., *The Breast Cancer Prevention Diet*, New York: Little Brown and Co., 1998; p. 93.

67. Schedlowski, M., et al., "Acute psychological stress increases plasma levels of cortisol, prolactin and thyroid stimulating hormone," *Life Sciences* 1992; 50: 1201–05.

68. "Drugs that cause sexual dysfunction: an update," *The Medical Letter* 1992; 34 (Issue 876).

69. Baghurst, P., et al., "Diet, prolactin and breast cancer," *Amer Jour Clin Nutr* 1992; 56: 943–49.

70. Ibid., Baghurst, p. 943–49.

71. Ibid., Baghurst, p. 943–49.

72. Panth, M., et al., "Effect of vitamin A supplementation on plasma progesterone and estradiol levels during pregnancy," *Int Jour Vit Nutr Res* 1991; p. 61.

73. Luck, M., et al., "Ascorbic acid and fertility," *Biol Reproduc* 1995; 52: 262–65.

74. Manvais-Jarvis, P., et al., "Progesterone and progestins: a general overview," *Progesterone and Progestins*, New York: Rave Press, 1983; p. 1–16.

75. Ibid., Vliet, p. 227.

76. Rouzier, N., "Estrogen and progesterone replacement," *Longevity and Preventive Medicine Symposium* 2002; p. 12.

77. Ibid., Bland, p. 66.

78. Ibid., Vliet, p. 25.

79. Ibid., Vliet, p. 96.

80. Sinatra, S., *Heart Sense for Women*. Washington, D.C.: LifeLine Press, 2000; p. 219.

81. Ottoson, U., et al., "Subfractions of high-density lipo-protein cholesterol during estrogen replacement therapy: A comparison between progestogens and natural progesterone," *Jour of Obstetrics and Gynec* 1985; 151: 746–50.

82. Ibid., Sinatra, p. 219.

83. Minshall, R., et al., "Ovarian steroid protection against coronary artery hyperreactivity in rhesus monkeys," *Jour Clin Endocrinol Metab* 1998; 83(2): 649–59.

84. Ottoson, U., et al., "Oral progesterone and estrogen/progestogen therapy; effects of natural and synthetic hormones on subfractions of HDL cholesterol and liver proteins," *ACTA Obstet Cynecol Scand* 1984; (Suppl), 127: 1–37.

85. Henderson, B., et al., "Estrogen replacement therapy and protection from acute MI," *Amer Jour Obstet Gynecol* 1988; 159: 312–17.

86. Lee, J., *What Your Doctor May Not Tell You About Menopause*. New York: Warner, 1996; p. 88.

87. Ibid., Rouzier, p. 13.

88. Ibid., Rouzier, p. 14.

89. Melton, L., et al., "Progestins reverse some of the effects of estrogen," *TEM* 2000; 11(2): 69–71.

90. Brownstein, D., *Overcoming Thyroid Disorders*. West Bloomfield, MI: Medical Alternatives Press, 2002; p. 113.

91. Ross, R., et al., "Effect of hormone replacement therapy on breast cancer risk: estrogen versus estrogen plus progestin," *Jour Natl Cancer Inst* 1992; (4): 328–32.

92. Schairer, C., et al., "Menopausal estrogen and estrogen-progestin replacement therapy and breast cancer risk," JAMA 2000; 283: 485–91.

93. Colditz, G., et al., "Use of estrogen plus progestin is associated with greater increase in breast cancer risk than estrogen alone," *Amer Jour Epidemiol* 1998; 147(Suppl): 64S.

94. Ibid., Laux, p. 75–6.

95. Majewska, M., et al., "Steroid hormone metabolites are barbiturate-like modulators of the GABA receptor," *Science* 1986; 232: 1004.

96. Clarkson, T., et al., "Conjugated equine estrogens alone, but not in combination with medroxyprogesterone acetate, inhibit aortic connective tissue remodeling after plasma lipid lowering in female monkeys," *Arterioscler Thromb Vasc Biol* 1998; 18(7): 1164–71.

97. Stefanick, M., et al., "Estrogen, progestogens and cardiovascular risk: review of PEPPI trial," *Jour Repro Med* 1999; 44(Suppl): 221–26.

98. Gerhard, M., et al., "Estradiol therapy combined wit progesteterone; endothelium-dependent vasodilation in postmenopausal women," *Circulation* 1998; 98(12): 1158–63.

99. Ibid., Rouzier, p. 13.

100. Ibid., Rouzier, p. 14.

101. Ibid., Sinatra, p. 219.

102. Ibid., Collins, p. 67.

103. Prior, J., et al., "Progesterone as a bone-tropic hormone," *Endocrine Reviews* 1990; 11:386–98.

104. Ibid., Vliet, p. 93.

105. Ibid., Clarkson, p. 1164–71.

106. Ibid., Bland, p. 57.

107. Khaw, K., et al., "Fasting plasma glucose levels and endogenous androgens in non-diabetic postmenopausal women," *Clin Sci* 1991; 80(3): 199–203.

108. Haffner, S., et al., "Endogenous sex hormones: impact on lipids, lipoproteins, and insulin," *Amer Jour Med* 1995; 98(1A): 40S–47S.

109. Kalkoff, R., et al., "Metabolic effects of progesterone," *Jour Obstect Gynecol* 1982; 142–6: 735–38.

110. Ibid., Vliet, p. 95.

111. Ibid., Vliet, p. 100.

112. Miodrg, A., et al., "Sex hormones and the female urinary tract," *Drugs* 1988; 36(4): 491–504.

113. Ibid., Vliet, p. 99.

114. Kalkoff, R., et al., "Metabolic effects of progesterone," *Jour Obstect Gynecol* 1982; 142–46: 735–38.

115. Ibid., Vliet, p. 97.

116. Ibid., Vliet, p. 98.

117. Persky, H., "Plasma testosterone level and sexual behavior of couples," *Arch Sex Behav* 1978; 7(3): 157–73.

118. Brincat, M., et al., "Sex hormones and skin collagen content in postmenopausal woman," *Brit Med Jour* 1983; 287(6402): 1337–38.

119. Sand, R., et al., "Exogenous androgens in postmenopausal women," *Amer Jour of Med* 1995; 98(1A).

120. Ibid., Vliet, p. 109.

121. Davis, S., et al., "Use of androgens in postmenopausal women," *Curr Opin Obstet Gynecol* 1997; 9(3): 177–180.

122. Surrel, P., et al., "Cardiovascular aspects of androgens in women," *Semin Repro Endocrin* 1998; 16(2): 121–28.

123. Shippen, E., *Testosterone Syndrome*. New York: M. Evans & Company, Inc., 1998; p. 152.

124. Schmidt, J., et al., "Other anti-androgens," *Dermatology* 1998; 196(1): 153–57.

125. *Nutrition and Healing Newsletter*, 1995; Vol. 11, No. 12.

126. Ibid., Laux, p. 119.

127. Springer-Verlag, S., *Testosterone: Action, Deficiency, Substitution*. Berlin, 1998; p. 299.

128. Ellison, P., et al., "Measurements of salivary progesterone," *Ann of the New York Acad of Sci* 1993; 694: 161–76.

129. Hofman, T., et al., "Steroid hormones in saliva," *Diagnostic Endocrinol Met* 1998; 16(9): 265–73.

130. Mandel, I., et al., "The diagnostic use of saliva," *Jour Oral Pathol Med* 1990; 19: 119–25.

131. Riad-Fahney, L., et al., "Steroids in saliva for assessing endocrine function," *Endocr Rev* 1982; 3(4): 367–95.

132. Vining, R., et al., "The measurements of hormones in saliva: possibility and pitfalls," *Jour of Steroid Biochem* 1987; 27: 81–94.

133. Vining, R., et al., "Hormones in saliva: mode of entry and consequent implications for clinical interpretation," *Clin Chemistry* 1983; 29(10): 1752–56.

Chapter 4: Male Hormones and Weight Loss

1. Korenman, S., et al., "Secondary hypogonadism in older men: Its relationship to impotence," *Jour Clin Endocrin Metab* 1990; 71: 963–69.

2. Shippen, E., *The Testosterone Syndrome*. New York, NY: M. Evans and Company, Inc., 1998; p. 21–27.

3. Malkin, C., et al., "The effect of testosterone replacement on endogenous inflammatory cytokines and lipid profiles in hypogonadal men," *Jour Clin Endocrinol Metab* 2004; 89(7): 3313–18.

4. Bhasin, S., "The dose-dependent effects of testosterone on sexual function and on muscle mass and function," *Mayo Clin Proc* 2000; Jan. 75(Suppl: S70–5).

5. Channer, K., et al., "Cardiovascular effects of testosterone: implications of the 'male menopause,'?" *Heart* 2003; 89(2): 121–22.

6. Webb, C., et al., "Effects of testosterone on coronary vasomotor regulation in men with coronary heart disease," *Circulation* 1999; 100(16): 1690–96.

7. Rothenberg, R., "Testosterone Replacement Therapy: Male Menopause," *Fellowship in Anti-Aging and Functional Medicine: Module I*, Las Vegas, NV, December 2006.

8. Boyanov, M., et al., "Testosterone supplementation in men with type 2 diabetes, visceral obesity and partial androgen deficiency," *Aging Male*. 2003; 6(1): 1–7.

9. Malkin C., et al., "Testosterone as a protective factor against atherosclerosis—immunomodulation and influence upon plaque development and stability," *Jour Endocrinolo* 2003; 78(3): 373–80.

10. Hak, A., et al., "Low levels of endogenous androgens increase the risk of atherosclerosis in elderly men: The Rotterdam Study," *Jour of Clin Endocrin & Metabol* 2002; 87(8): 3632–39.

11. Muller, M., et al., "Endogenous sex hormones and progression of carotid atherosclerosis in elderly men," *Circulation* 2004; 109(17): 2074–79.

12. Alexander, G., et al., "Androgen-behavior correlations in hypogonadal men and eugonadal men. II. Cognitive abilities," *Hormones and Behavior* 1998; 33(2): 85–94.

13. Barrett-Connor, E., et al., "Endogenous sex hormones and cognitive function in older men," *Jour Clin Endocrin Metabol* 1999; 84(10): 3681–85.

14. Moffat, S., et al., "Long-term measures of free testosterone predict regional cerebral blood flow patterns in elderly men," *Neurobiol Aging* 2006; May 11.

15. Burris, A., et al., "A long-term, prospective study of the physiology and behavioral effects of hormone replacement in untreated hypogonadal men," *Jour Androl* 1992; 13(4): 297–304.

16. Gouras, G., et al., "Testosterone reduces neuronal secretion of Alzheimer's beta-amyloid peptides," *Proc Nat Acad Sci USA* 97(3): 1202–05.

17. Hogervorst, E., et al., "Low free testosterone is an independent risk factor for Alzheimer's disease," *Exp Gerontol* 2004; 39(11–12): 1633–39.

18. Tan, R., "A pilot study on the effects of testosterone in hypogonadal aging male patients with Alzheimer's disease," *Aging Male* 2003; 6(1): 13–7.

19. Baran, D., et al., "Effect of testosterone therapy on bone formation in an osteoporotic hypogonadal male," *Calified Tissue Res* 1978; 26: 103–06.

20. Murphy, S., et al., "Sex hormones and bone mineral density in elderly men," *Bone Mineral* 1993; 20: 133–40.

21. Jackson, J., et al., "Testosterone deficiency as a risk factor for hip fractures in men: a case-control study," *Amer Jour of Med Sci* 1992; 304: 4–8.

22. +++++++++

23. Ibid., Shippen, p. 50.

24. Ibid., Shippen, p. 211–12.

25. Ibid., Shippen, p. 212.

Chapter 5: Pregnenolone and Weight Loss

1. Roberts, E., et al., "Pregnenolone—from Selye to Alzheimer's and a model of the pregnenolone sulfate finding site on the GABA receptor," *Biochemical Pharm* 1995; 49(1): 1–16.

2. Yanick, P., *Prohormone Nutrition*. Montclair, N.J.: Longevity Institute International, 1998; p. 358.

Chapter 6: Insulin and Weight Loss

1. Vliet, E., *Women Weight and Hormones*. New York: Evans & Company, 2001; p. 154.

2. Ibid., Vliet, p. 154.

3. Schwarzbein, D., *The Schwarzbein Principle II*. Deerfield Beach, FL: Health Communications, Inc., 2002.

4. Brewerton, T., et al., "Toward a unified theory of serotonin dysregulation in eating and related disorders," Psychoneuroendocrin 1995; 20: 561–90.

5. Houston, M., "The metabolic syndrome: pathophysiology, diagnosis, clinical aspects, prevention and nonpharmacologic treatment: emphasis on lifestyle modifications, nutrition, nutritional supplements, vitamins, minerals, antioxidants, weight management and exercise," JANA 2005; 8(2):7.

6. Foster-Powell, K., et al., "International tables of glycemic index," *Amer Jour of Clin Nutrition* 1995; 62: 871S–893S.

7. Ibid., p. 871–935.

8. Ibid., p. 871–935.

9. Pereira M., et al., *JAMA* 2004; 292(20): 2482–90.

10. Raikkonen, K., et al., "Psychosocial stress and the insulin resistance syndrome," *Metabolism* 1996; 45: 1533–38.

11. Nilsson, P., et al., "Adverse effects of psychosocial stress on gonadal function and insulin levels in middle-aged males," *Jour Inter Med* 1995; 237: 479–86.

12. Friedman, T., et al., "Carbohydrate and lipid metabolism in endogenous hypercortisolism: shared features with metabolic syndrome X and NIDDM," *Endocr Jour* 1996; 43: 645–55.

13. Smith, P., *Vitamins: Hype or Hope*. Traverse City, MI: Healthy Living Books, 2004.

14. Kaczmar, T., "Herbal support for diabetes management," *Clinical Nutrition Insights* 1998; 6(8): 1–4.

15. Marles, F., et al., "Antidiabetic plants and their active constituents: an update," *Protocol Jour Nat Med* 1996; 85: 111.

16. Baskaran, K., et al., "Antidiabetic effect of a leaf extract form Gymnema sylvestre in non-insulin-dependent diabetes mellitus patients," *Jour Ethnopharmacol* 1990; 30: 295–305.

17. Sharma, R., et al., "Effect of fenugreek seeds on blood glucose and serum insulin responses in human subjects," *Nutr Res* 1986; 6: 1353–64.

18. Madar, Z., et al., "Glucose-lowering effect of fenugreek in non-insulin dependent diabetics," *Eur Jour Clin Nutr* 1988; 42: 51–4.

19. Elder, C., "Ayurveda for diabetes mellitus: a review of the biomedical literature," *Alternative Therapies* 2004; 10(1): 44–50.

20. Stivastava, Y., et al., "Antidiabetic and adaptogenic properties of Momordica charantia extract: an experimental and clinical evaluation," *Phytotherapy Res* 1993; 7: 285–89.

21. Berrio, L., et al., "Insulin activity: stimulatory effects of cinnamon and Brewer's yeast as influenced by albumin," *Horm Res* 1992; 37: 225–29.

Chapter 7: Thyroid Hormone Dysfunction and Weight Loss

1. Horst, C., et al., "Rapid stimulation of hepatic oxygen consumption by 3,5-di-iodo-1-thyrooninne," *Biochem Journ* 1989; 261: 945–50.

2. Rouzier, N., "Estrogen and progesterone replacement," *Longevity and Preventive Medicine Symposium*. 2002; p. 8.

3. Brownstein, D., *Overcoming Thyroid Disorders*. West Bloomfield, MI: Medical Alternatives Press, 2002, p. 8.

4. Ibid., Rouzier, p. 3.

5. Hale, A., et al., "Subclinical hypothyroidism is an independent risk factor for atherosclerosis and MI in elderly women: The Rotterdam study," *Ann Inter Med* 2000; 132: 270–78.

6. Nishiyama, S., et al., "Zinc supplementation alters thyroid hormone metabolism in disabled patients with zinc deficiency," *Jour Amer Coll Nutr* 1994; 13: 62–7.

7. Meinhold, H., et al., "Effects of selenium and iodine deficiency on iodothyronine deiodinases in brain, thyroid and peripheral tissue," *JAMA* 1992; 19: 8–12.

8. Berry, M., et al., "The role of selenium in thyroid hormone action," *Endocrine Rev* 1992; 13: 207–20.

9. Kohrle, J., et al., "The deiodinase family; selenoenzymes regulating thyroid hormone availability and action," *Cell Mol Life Sci* 2000; 57: 1853–63.

10. Ibid., Brownstein, p. 27.

11. Brownstein, D., *The Miracle of Natural Hormones*. West Bloomfield, MI: Medical Alternatives Press, 1998; p. 11.

12. Rouzier, N., "Thyroid replacement therapy," Longevity and Preventive Medicine Symposium 2002, p. 16.

13. Pansini, F., "Effect of the hormonal contraception on serum reverse triiodothyronine levels," *Gynecol Obstet Invest* 1987; 23: 133.

14. Ibid., Pansini, p. 133.

15. Vliet, E., *Women Weight and Hormones*. New York: Evans & Co., 2001; p. 127.

16. Divi, R., et al., "Anti-thyroid isoflavones from soybean: isolation, characterization, and mechanism of action," *Biochem Pharmacol* 1997; 54: 10, 1087–96.

17. Ibid., Vliet, p. 128.

18. Nishida, M., et al., "Direct evidence for the presence of methylmercury bound in the thyroid and other organs obtained from mice give methylmercury; differentiation of free and bound methylmercuries in biological materials determined by volatility of methylmercury," *Chem Pharm Bull* 1990; 38(5): 1412–13.

19. Rachman, B., "Managing endocrine imbalance; autoimmune-induced thyroidopathy and chronic fatigue syndrome," *Functional Medicine Approaches to Endocrine Disturbances of Aging*. Gig Harbor, Washington: The Institute for Functional Medicine, 2001, p. 226.

20. Beard, J., "Impaired thermoregulation and thyroid function in iron deficiency anemia," *Amer Jour Clin Nutr* 1990; 52: 813–19.

21. Lenon, d., et al., "Diet and exercise training effects on resting metabolic rate," *Int. Jour Obesity* 1985; 9: 39–47.

22. Vunevicius, R., et al., "Effects of thyroxine as compared with thyroxine plus triiodothyroxine in patients with hypothyroidism," *NEJM* 1999; 340: 424.

23. Ibid., p. 424–29.

24. Ibid., Brownstein, *Overcoming Thyroid Disorders*, p. 37.

25. Fed Register. August 14, 1997; 62(157).

26. Ibid, Brownstein, *Overcoming Thyroid Disorders*.

Chapter 8: Detoxification and Weight Loss

1. *The Importance of Detoxification*. Advanced Nutritional Publications, Inc., 2002.

2. Ibid., *The Importance of Detoxification*.

3. Ibid., *The Importance of Detoxification*.

4. Ibid., *The Importance of Detoxification*.

5. Lazarou, J., et al., "Incidence of adverse drug reaction in hospitalized patients," *JAMA* 1998; 279(15): 1200–05.

6. Genova Diagnostic Laboratory.

7. Hanaway, P. "Optimizing Gut Function," *Module III, Fellowship in Anti-Aging and Functional Medicine*, April 2006, Orlando, Florida.

8. Ibid., p. 1–61.

9. Sahley, B., *Heal with Amino Acids and Nutrients*. San Antonio Texas: Pain & Stress Publications, 2000.

Chapter 9: Inflammation and Weight Loss

1. Houston, M., "The metabolic syndrome: pathophysiology, diagnosis, clinical aspects, prevention and nonpharmacologic treatment: Emphasis on lifestyle modifications, nutrition, nutritional supplements, vitamins, minerals, antioxidants, weight management and exercise," *JANA* 2005; 8(2): 28.

2. Ibid., Houston, p. 28.

3. Ibid., Houston, p. 28.

4. Guilliams, T., "Managing chronic inflammation: natural solutions," *The Standard* 2006; 7(2): 3.

5. Nicklas, B., et al., "Behavioral treatments for chronic systemic inflammation: effects of dietary weight loss and exercise training," *CMAJ* 2005; 72(9): 1199–1204.

6. Dietrich, M., et al., "The effect of weight loss on a stable biomarker of inflammation, c-reactive protein," *Nutrition Reviews* 2005; 63(1): 22–8.

7. Qi, L., et al., "Whole-grain, bran, and cereal fiber intakes and markers of systemic inflammation in diabetic women," *Diabetes Care* 2006; 29(2): 207–11.

8. Lu, S., et al., "Relation between a diet with a high glycemic load and plasma concentrations of high sensitivity c-reactive protein in middle-aged women," *Amer Jour Clin Nutr* 2002; 75(3): 492–98.

9. Rakel, D., et al., "Inflammation: nutritional, botanical, and mind-body influences," *Southern Med Journ* 2005; 98(3): 303–09.

10. Ibid., Nicklas, p. 1199–1204.

11. Esposito, K., et al., *JAMA* 2003; 289: 1799–1804.+++++++

12. Cesarri, M., et al., Amer Jour Clin Nutr 2005; 82: 428–34.

13. Bruunsgaard, H., "Physical activity and modulation of systemic low-level inflammation," *Jour Leukocyte Biol* 2005; 78: 819–35.

14. Miller, G., et al., "Chronic psychological stress and the regulation of pro-inflammatory cytokines: a glucocorticoid-resistance model," *Health Psychology* 2002; 21(6): 531–41.

15. Challem, J., *The Inflammation Syndrome*. Hoboken, N.J.: John Wiley & Sons, Inc., 2003, p. 16–17.

16. Lerman, R., "Nutrients as biological response modifiers: fatty acids and inflammation," *Applying Functional Medicine in Clinical Practice*. Gig Harbor, Washington: Institute for functional Medicine, 2002; p. 33.

17. Schmidt, M., Brain-Building Nutrition: *The Healing Power of Fats and Oils*. Berkeley, CA: Frog, Ltd., 2001.

18. Erasmus, Udo, *Fats That Heal, Tats That Kill*. Burnaby, BC, Canada: Alive Books, 1993.

19. Colgan, M., *The New Nutrition*. Vancouver, British Columbia, Canada: Apple Publishing, 1995; p. 146–49.

20. Bland, J., *Clinical Nutrition: A Functional Approach*. Gig Harbor, Washington: Institute for Functional Medicine, 1999; p. 71–95.

21. Ibid., Erasmus, p. 21–22.

22. Lerman, R., "The essential fatty acids in psychiatric and neurological dysfunction," Brain Biochemistry and nutrition," Gig Harbor Washington: The Institute for Functional Medicine, 2002; p. 65.

23. Goodman, J., *The Omega Solution*. Roseville, CA: Prima Publishing, 2001; p. 47.

24. Ibid., Bland, p. 279.

25. Ibid., Lerman, p. 1.

26. Ibid., Colgan, p. 144.

27. Ibid., Colgan, p. 145.

28. Ibid., Colgan, p. 145.

29. Ibid., Schmidt, p. 76.

30. Blum, S., et al., "Effect of a Mediterranean meal on postprandial carotenoids, paramonase and c-reactive protein levels," *Ann Nutr Metabol* 2006; 0(1): 20–4.

31. Esposito, K., et al., "Effect of a Mediterranean-style diet on endothelial dysfunction and makers of vascular inflammation in the metabolic syndrome. A randomized trial," *JAMA* 2004; 292(12): 1440–46.

32. Greenberg, A., et al., "Obesity and the role of adipose tissue in inflammation and metabolism," *Amer Jour Clin Nutr* 2006; 83(2): 461S–465S.

33. Rountree, R., "Immune dysfunction and inflammation, Part II," *Applying Functional Medicine in Clinical Practice*. Gig Harbor, Washington: The Institute for Functional Medicine, 2002; p. 1–30.

34. Ibid., Rountree, p. 21.

35. Ibid., Rountree, p. 21.

36. Ibid., Rountree, p. 24.

37. Ibid., Rountree, p. 25.

Chapter 10: Sleep Deprivation and Weight Loss

1. Goldman, R., Klatz, R., *Sleep: Essential for Optimal Health*. Chicago: American Academy of Anti-Aging Medicine, 2003, p. 6

2. ++++*Jour Clin Endocrin Metab* 2001; 86(8): 3787–94.

3. Ibid, Goldman, p. 5.

4. +++++Spiegel, ++et. al., ++++*Jour Clin Endocrin Metab* 2004; 89(11): 5762–71.

5. Ibid., Goldman, p. 19.

6. Brandenberger, G., et al., "Effect of sleep deprivation on overall 24 hour growth-hormone secretion," *Lancet* 2000; 356(9230): 1408.

7. LaValle, J., "Current Concepts in Metabolic Regulation: The Role of Nutrients and Novel Agents," *Module IV, Fellowship in Anti-Aging and Functional Medicine*, Detroit, MI, October 2006.

8. Spiegel, K., et al., "Impact of sleep on metabolic and endocrine function," *Lancet* 1999; 354(9188): 1435–39.

9. Schmidt, *Tired of Being Tired*, p. 204–07.++++++++++++++++

10. Edling, C., et al., "Occupational exposure to organic solvents as a cause of sleep apnea," *Br Jour Indust Med* 1993; 50: 276–79.

11. Steiger, A., et al., "Effects of hormones on sleep," *Horm Res* 1998; 49(3–4): 125–30.

12. James, S., et al., "Melatonin administration in insomnia." *Neuropsychopharmacology* 1990; 3(1): 19–23.

13. Vliet, E., *Women, Weight and Hormones*. New York: M. Evans & Company, 2001; p. 149.

14. Brzezinski, A., et al., "Melatonin in humans," *NEJM* 1997; 336(3): 186–95.

15. Bland, J., "Obesity and endocrine signaling," *Improving Intercellular Communication in Managing Chronic Illness*. Gig Harbor Washington: Health Comm International, Inc., 1999, p. 124.

16. Lieberman, S., *The Real Vitamin and Mineral Book*. New York: Avery Publishing, 1997; p. 216.

17. Foss-Morgan, R., *Hormone Replacement Therapy*. Haddonfield, New Jersey: Anti-Aging and Longevity Medical Center of Haddonfield, 2000.

18. Ibid., Bland, p. 125.

19. Poeggeler, B., et al., "Melatonin—a highly potent endogenous radical scavenger and electron donor: new aspects of the oxidation chemistry of this indole accessed in vitro," *Ann NY Acad Sci* 1994; 738: 419–21.

20. Tan, D., et al., "Melatonin: a potent endogeneous hydroxyl radical scavenger," *Endocrine Jour* 1993; 1: 57–60.

21. Ibid., Lieberman, p. 216.

22. Ibid., Lieberman, p. 216.

23. Ibid., Lieberman, p. 217.

24. Ibid., Foss-Morgan.

25. Ibid., Lieberman, p. 217.

26. Ibid., Bland, p. 127.

27. Ibid., Vliet, p. 150.

28. Ibid., Brzezinski, p. 186–95.

29. Chesson, A., etal., "Current trends in the management of insomnia," *Emergency Med April,* 2002; p. 11–18.

30. Ibid., Goldman.

31. Garfinkel, D., et al., "Improvement of sleep quality in elderly people by controlled-release melatonin," *Lancet* 1995; 346(8974): 541–44.

32. Haimov, I., et al., "Melatonin replacement therapy of elderly insomnia," *Sleep* 1995; 18(7): 598–603.

33. Hornyak, M., et al., "Magnesium therapy for periodic leg movements-related insomnia and restless legs syndrome: an open pilot study," *Sleep* 1998; 21: 501–05.

34. James, S., et al., "Melatonin administration in insomnia," *Neuropsychopharm* 1990; 3(1): 19–23.

35. Pastora, J., et al., "Flavonoids from lemon balm (Melissa officinalis L., Lamiaceae)," *Acta Pol Pharm* 2002; 59(2): 139–43.

36. Speroni, E., et al., "Neuropharmacologicial activity of extracts from Passiflora incarnate," *Planta Med* 1988; 488–91.

Chapter 11: Exercise and Weight Loss

1. Anonymous, "Prostaglandins, brown fat, and weight loss," *Med Hypoth* 1989; 28:13.

2. Grimm, J., et al., "Interaction of physical activity and diet: implications for insulin-glucose dynamics," *Public Health Nutr* 1999; 2: 363–68.

3. Ivy, J., et al., "Role of exercise training in the prevention and treatment of insulin resistance and non-insulin-dependent-diabetes mellitus," *Sports Med* 1997; 24: 321–60.

4. Lehmann, R., et al., "Loss of abdominal fat and improvement of the cardiovascular risk profile by regular moderate exercise training in patients with NIDDM," *Diabetologia* 1995; 38: 1313–19.

5. Horber, F., et al., "Effect of regular physical training on age-associated alteration of body composition in men," *Eur Jour Clin Invest* 1996; 26: 279–85.

6. Hughes, V., et al., "Exercise increases muscle GLUT-4 levels and insulin action in subjects with impaired glucose tolerance," *Amer Jour Physiol* 1993; 264: E855–E862.

7. Walberg, J., et al., "Aerobic exercise and resistance weight-training during weight reduction. Implications for obese persons and athletes," *Sports Med* 1989; 7: 343–56.

Chapter 12: Fiber Intake and Weight Loss

1. Anderson, J., et al., "Dietary fiber: diabetes and obesity," *Amer Jour Gsteroenterol* 1986; 81:898–906.

2. Burke, V., et al., "Dietary protein and soluble fiber reduce ambulatory blood pressure in treatment of hypertensives," *Hypertension* 2001; 38(4): 821–26.

3. Anderson, J., et al., "High-fiber diets for diabetic and hypertriglyceridemic patients," *Can med Assoc Jour* 1980; 123: 975.

4. Sprecher, D., et al., "Efficacy of psyllium in reducing serum cholesterol levels in hypercholesterolemic patients on high-or-low-fat diets," *Ann Inter Med* 1993; 119: 545–54.

5. Rodriguez-Moran, M., et al., "Lipid and glucose-lowering efficacy of plantago psyllium in type II diabetes," *Jour Diabetes Complications* 1998; 12: 273–78.

6. Landin, K., et la., "Guar gum improves insulin sensitivity, blood lipids, blood pressure, and fibrinolysis in healthy men," *Amer Jour Clin Nutr* 1992; 56: 1061–65.

7. Klatz, R., and Goldman, R., *7 Anti-Aging Secrets*. Chicago, IL: Elite Sports Medicine Publications, 1996, 52–53, 57.

8. Houston, M, *What Your Doctor May Not Tell You About Hypertension*. New York: Warner Books, Inc., 2003, p. 147–48.

9. Ibid., Klatz, p. 52–53, 57.

10. Ibid., Houston, p. 147–48.

Chapter 13: Water and Weight Loss

1. Batmanghelidj, B., *Your Body's Many Cries for Water.* Vienna, VA: Global Health Solutions, 1992.

Chapter 14: Yeast Infections and Weight Loss

1. Crook, W., *The Yeast Connection Handbook*. Jackson, TN: Professional Books, Inc., 2002.

2. Appleton, *Stopping Inflammation*. Garden City Park, NY: Square One Publishers, 2005.

3. Ibid., Crook, p. 1–5.

4. Ibid., Appleton, p. 69–72.

5. Ponikau, J., et al., "The diagnosis and incidence of allergic fungal sinusitis," *Mayo Clinic Proceedings 1999*; 74: 877–84.

6. Ibid., Crook, p. 32, 34, 49.

7. Ibid., Crook, p. 8.

8. Ibid., Appleton, p. 69.

9. Ibid., Crook, p. 129–33.

10. Ibid., Crook, p. 105–06.

11. Ibid., Crook, p. 98.

Chapter 15: Neurotransmitters and Weight Loss

1. von Bohlen und Halback, O., *Neurotransmitters and Neuromodultors.* 2002.++++++++++

2. Nester, E., *Molecular NeuroPharmacology*. New York: McGraw-Hill, 2001.

3. LeDoux, J., *Synaptic Self: Our Brains Become Who We Are.* New York: Penguin Books, 2002.

4. Sahley, B., *The Anxiety Amino Acid.* San Antonio, Texas: Pain & Stress Publications, 1999.

5. Klatz, R., *The New Anti-Aging Revolution,* North Bergen, NJ: Basic Health Publications, 2003; p. 236.

6. Waagepetersen, H., et al., "The GABA paradox: multiple roles as a metabolite, neurotransmitter and neurodifferentiative agent," *Jour Neurochem* 1999; 73(4):1335–42.

7. Ibid., Sahley, p. 16.

8. Ibid., Klatz, p. 236.

9. Meguid, M., et al., "Hypothalamic dopamine and serotonin in the regulation of food intake," *Nutrition* 2000; 16(10):843–57.

10. Hamon, M., et al., "Role of serotonin and other neuroactive molecules in the physiopathogenesis of migraine," *Pathol Bio* (Paris) 2000; 48(7): 619–29.

11. Sahley, B., *Healing with Amino Acids and Nutrients*. San Antonio, Texas: Pain & Stress Publications, 2000; p. 50–51.

12. Ibid., Klatz, p. 256–57.

13. Bond, A., et al., "Tryptophan depletion increases aggression in women during the premenstrual phase," *Psychopharm* (Berl) 2001; 156(4): 477–80.

14. Ibid., Sahley, p. 52.

15. Ibid., Sahley, p. 49.

16. den Boer, J., et al., "Behavior, neuroendocrine, and biochemical effects of 5-hydroxytryptophan administration in panic disorder," *Psychiatry Res* 1990; 31: 267–78.

17. Ribeiro, C., et al., "5-hydroxytryptophan in the prophylaxis of chronic tension-type headache: a double-blind, random, placebo-controlled study for the Portuguese Head Society," *Headache* 2000; 40: 451–56.

18. Birdshell, T., "5–hydroxytryptophan: A clinically-effective serotonin precursor," *Alt Med* Rev 1998; 3: 271–78.

19. Ibid., Klatz, p. 241.

20. Ibid., Sahley, p. 40.

21. Ibid., Sahley, p. 40.

22. Ibid., Klatz, p. 242.

23. Ibid., Klatz, p. 252–53.

24. Ibid., Sahley, 48.

25. Kendler, B., et al., "Taurine: an overview of its role in preventive medicine," *Prev Med* 1989; 18(1): 70–100.

26. Huxtable, R., et al., "Physiologic actions of taurine," *Physiol Rev* 1992; 72: 101–63.

27. Chapman, R., et al., "Taurine and the heart," *Cardiovasc Res* 1993; 27(3): 358–63.

29. Redmond, H., et al., "Immunonutrition: the role of taurine," *Nutrition* 1998; 14(7–8): 599–604.

30. Crayhon, R. "Aging well in the 21st century," *Seminar* 2002.

31. Gaby, A., *Nutritional Therapy in Medical Practice*. Carlisle, PA: Nutrition Seminars, 2003; p. 58.

32. Dawson, R., "An age-related decline in striatal taurine is correlated with a loss of dopaminergic markers," *Brain Res Bull* 199; 48: 319–24.

33. Birdsall, T., "Therapeutic applications of taurine," *Altern Med Rev* 1998; 3: 128–36.

34. Kumata, K., et al., "Restoration of endothelium-dependant relaxation in both hypercholesterolemic and diabetics by chronic taurine," *Eur Jour Pharmacol* 1996; 303: 47–53.

35. Lombardini, J., et al., "Taurine retinal function," *Brain Res Rev* 1991; 16(2): 151–69.

36. Zackheim, H., et al., "Taurine and psoriasis," *Jour Invest Dermatol* 1968; 50(23): 277–30.

37. Nakagawa, M., et al., "Antihypertensive effect of taurine on the salt-induced hypertension," *Adv Exp Med Biol* 1994; 359: 197–206.

38. Fujita, T., et al., "Hypotensive effect of taurine, possible involvement of the sympathetic nervous system and endogenous opiates," *Jour Clin Invest* 1988; 82(3): 993–97.

39. Desai, T., et al., "Taurine deficiency after intensive chemotherapy and/or radiation," *Amer Jour Clin Nutr* 1992; 55(3): 708–11.

40. Collins, B., "Plasma and urinary taurine in epilepsy," *Clin Chem* 1988; 34(4): 671–75.

41. Ibid., Klatz, p. 231.

42. Sinatra, S., *Heart Sense For Women*. Washington, D.C.: LifeLine Press, 2000; p. 150.

43. Efron, D., et al., "Role of arginine in immunonutrition," *Jour Gastroenterol* 2000; 35(suppl 12): 20–3.

44. Ibid., Sahley, p. 23–4.

45. Siani, A., et al., "Blood pressure and metabolic changes during dietary L-arginine supplementation in humans," *Amer Jour Hypertens* 2000; 13(5, Pt. 1): 547–51.

46. Ibid., Klatz, p. 231.

47. Great Smokies Diagnostic Laboratory Interpretive Guidelines for Amino Acid Analysis.

48. Lee, Z, et al., "Urinary epinephrine and norepinephrine interrelations with obesity, insulin, and the metabolic syndrome in Hong Kong Chinese," *Metabolsim* 2001; 50(2): 135–43.

49. Rosenbaum, M., et al., "Effects of changes in body weight on carbohydrate metabolism, catecholamine excretion, and thyroid function," *Amer Jour Clin Nutr* 2000; 71(6): 1421–32.

50. Delgado, P., et al., "Role of norepinephrine in depression," *Jour Clin Psychiatry* 2000; 61: (Suppl 1): 5–12.

51. Shabert, J., *The Ultimate Nutrient Glutamine*. Garden City Par, New York: Avery Publishing Group, 1994; p. 2.

52. Maskovitz, B., et al., "Glutamine metabolism and utilization: relevance to major problems in health care," *Pharmacol Res* 1994; 30(1): 61–71.

53. Ibid., Sahley, p. 35–37.

54. Ibid., Klatz, p. 238.

55. Keast, D., et al., "Depression of plasma glutamine concentration after exercise stress and its possible influence on the immune system," *Med Jour Aust* 1995; 162(1): 15–8.

56. Nurjhan, N., et al., "Glutamine: a major gluconeogenic precursor and vehicle for interorgan carbon transport in man," *Jour Clin Invest* 1995; 95(1): 272–77.

57. Peck, L., et al., "Glutamine should be figured into inflammatory bowel disease formulations," *Family Practice News* 1994; June, p. 22.

58. Welbourne, T., et al., "Increased plasma bicarbonate and growth hormone after an oral glutamine load," *Amer Jour Clin Nutr* 1995; 61(5): 1058–61.

59. Ibid., Klatz, p. 238.

60. Ibid., Klatz, p. 240.

61. Blaylock, R., *Excitotoxins: The Taste That Kills*. Santa Fe, NM: Health Press, 1997; p. 34.

Chapter 16: The Science Behind Food Addictions

1. Stahl, S., et al., "The psychopharmacology of sex, Part 1: neurotransmitters and the 3 phases of the human sexual response," *Jour Clin Psy* 2001; 62: 80–1.

2. Koehler, P., et al., "High pressure liquid chromatographic analysis of tyramine, phenylethylamine and tryptamine in sausage, cheese, and chocolate," *Jour of Food Sci* 1978; 43: 1245–47.

3. Di Tomaso, E., et al., "Brain cannabinoids in chocolate," *Nature* 1996; 382: 677–78.

4. Shah, N., et al., "Effects of milk-derived bioactives: an overview," *Brit Jour Nutr* 2000; 84 (Suppl 1): S3–S10.

5. Chan, J., et al., "Dairy products, calcium, and prostate cancer risk in the Physicians' Health Study," *Amer Jour Clin Nutr* 2001; 74: 549–54.

6. Cella, F., et al., "Effects of dietary restriction on serum leptin concentration in obese women," *Int Jour Obes* 1999; 23: 494–97.

7. Wang, G., et al., "Brain dopamine and obesity," *Lancet* 2001; 357: 354–57.

8. Barnard, N., *Breaking the Food Seduction*. New York: St. Martin's Press, 2003.

Chapter 17: Nutrients That Aid in Weight Loss

1. Hart, C., *The Insulin-Resistance Diet*. Chicago: Contemporary Books, 2001, p. 91.

2. Colgan, M., *The New Nutrition*. Vancover, B.C., Canada: Apple Publishing, 1995, p. 103.

3. Lieberman, S., *The Real Vitamin ad Mineral Book*. New York: Avery Publishing Group, 1997, p. 54.

4. Bateman, J., et al., "Possible toxicity of herbal remedies," *Scottish Med Jour* 1998; 4: 7–15.

5. Ibid., Colgan, p. 104.

6. Murray, C., et al., "Alternative projections of mortality and disability by cause 1990–2020: global burden of disease study," *Lancet* 1997; 349: 1498–1504.

7. Meletis, C., *Interactions Between Drugs and Natural Medicines*. Sandy, Oregon: Electric Medical Publications, 1999.

8. Fuhr, U., et al., "Drug interactions with grapefruit juice, extent, probable mechanism, and clilnical relevance," *Drug Sci* 1998; 18: 251–72.

9. Ibid., Meletis.

10. Ibid., Colgan.

11. Ibid., Liberman.

12. Ulene, A., *Dr. Art Ulene=s Complete Guide to Vitamins, Minerals, and Herbs*. New York: Avery Publishing, 2000.

13. Ibid., Colgan, p. 14.

14. Ibid., Lieberman, p. 21.

15. Ibid., Lieberman, p. 22.

16. Galland. L., "Person-centered diagnosis and chronic fatigue," *Metabolic Energy, Messenger Molecules, and Chronic Illness: The Functional Perspective*. Gig Harbor, Washington: Institute for Functional Medicine, 2000, p. 326.

17. Moya-Camarena, S., et al., "Conjugated linoleic acid is a potent naturally occurring ligand and activator of PPAR," *Jour Lipid Res* 1999; 40: 1426–33.

18. Riserus, U., et al., "Conjugated linoleic acid (CLA) reduced abdominal adipose tissue in obese middle-aged men with signs of metabolic syndrome: a randomized controlled trial," *Int Jour Obes Related Metab Disord* 2001; 25(8): 1129–35.

19. Blankson, H., et al., "Conjugated linoleic acid reduces body fat mass in overweight and obese humans," *Jour Nutr* 2000; 130(12): 2943–48.

20. Pariza, M., et al., "Conjugated dienoic derivatives of linolic acid: a new class of anticarcinogerns," *Med Oncol Tumor Pharmacother* 1990; 7(2–3): 169–71.

21. Belury, M., et al., "Conjugated dienoic linoleate: a polyunsaturated fatty acid with unique chemoprotective properties," **Nur Res** 1995; 53(4 Pt. 1): 83–9.

22. Epstein, F., et al., "Glucose transporters and insulin action: implication for insulin resistance and diabetes mellitus," *NEJM* 1999; 341(4): 248–57.

23. Ryder, J., et al., "Isomer-specific antidiabetic properties of conjugated linoleic acid. Improve glucose tolerance skeletal muscle insulin action, and UCP-2 gene expression," *Diabetes* 2001; 50: 1149–57.

24. Doyle, L., et al., "Scientific forum explores CLA knowledge," *Inform* 1998; 9(1): 69.

25. Crayhon, R., *The Carnitine Miracle*. New York: M. Evans and Company, Inc., 1998.

26. Sahley, B., *Heal with Amino Acids and Nutrients*. San Antonio Texas: Pain & Stress Publications, 2000, p. 28–31.

27. Klatz, R., *The New Anti-Aging Revolution*. North Bergen, New Jersey: Basic Health Publications, 2003, p. 229.

28. Bland, J., *Clinical Nutrition: A Functional Approach*. Gig Harbor, Washington: Institute for Functional Medicine, 1999, p. 50–1.

29. Bland, J., *Applying Functional Medicine in Clinical Practice*. Gig Harbor, Washington: Institute for Functional Medicine, 2002, p. 16.

30. Tanphaichitr, V., et al., "Carnitine metabolism and carnitine deficiency," *Nutr* 1993; 9: 246–54.

31. Gaby, A., *Nutritional Therapy in Medical Practice*. Carlisle, PA: Nutrition Seminars, 2003, p. 50.

32. Young, G., *Ningxia Wolfberry: The Ultimate Superfood*. Orem, Utah: Essential Science Publishing, 2006, p. 29.

33. Ibid., p. 172.

34. Ibid., p. 172.

35. Berkey, C., et al., "Milk, dairy fat, dietary calcium, and weight gain: a longitudinal study of adolescents," *Arch Pediatr Adolesc Med* 2005; 159(6): 543–50.

36. Moreira, P., et al., "Dietary calcium and body mass index in Portuguese children," *Eur Jour Clin Nutr* 2005; May 25.

37. Ibid., Young, p. 172.

Conclusion

1. Champagne, C., et al., "Energy intake and energy expenditure: a controlled study comparing dietitians and non-dietitians," *Jour Amer Diet Assoc* 2002; 102(10): 1428–32.

2. Hyman, M., "Systems biology: the gut-brain-fat cell connection and obesity," *Alt Ther* 2006; 12(1): 10–16.

3. Rosenbaum, M., "Obesity," *NEJM* 1997; 337(6): 396–407.

4. Bray, G., et al., "Consumption of high-fructose corn syrup in beverages may play a role in the epidemic of obesity," (published correction appears in *Amer Jour Clin Nutr* 2004; 80(4): 1090), *Amer Jour Clin Nutr* 2004; 79(4): 537–43.

5. Ibid., Hyman, p. 10–16.

6. Lavin, J., et al., "The effect of sucrose-and aspartame-sweetened drinks on energy intake, hunger, and food choice of female, moderately restrained eaters," *Int Jour Obes Relat Metab Disord* 1997; 21: 37–42.

7. Tordoff, M., et al., "Oral stimulation with aspartame increases hunger," *Physiol Behav* 1990; 47: 555–59.

8. Farshchi, H., et al., "Deleterious effects of omitting breakfast on insulin sensitivity and fasting lipid profiles in healthy lean women," *Amer Jour Clin Nutr* 2005; 81(2): 388–96.

9. Farshchi, H., et al., "Beneficial metabolic effects of regular meal frequency on dietary thermogenesis, insulin sensitivity, and fasting lipid profiles in healthy obese women," *Amer Jour Clin Nutr* 2005; 81(1): 16–24.

10. Jenkins, D., et al., "Nibbling versus gorging: metabolic advances of increased meal frequency," *NEJM* 1989; 321: 929–34.

11. Pereira, M., et al., "Effects of a low-glycemic load diet on resting energy expenditure and heart disease risk factors during weight loss," *JAMA* 2004; 292(20): 2482–90.

12. Ludwig, D., et al., "Dietary fiber, weight gain, and cardiovascular disease risk factors in young adults," *JAMA* 1999; 282(16): 1539–46.

13. Ibid., Hyman, p. 15.

14. Vuksan, V., et al., "Beneficial effects of viscous dietary fiber from Konjac-mannan in subjects with the insulin resistance syndrome: results of a controlled metabolic trial," *Diabetes Care* 2000; 23(1): 9–14.

15. Juntunen, K., et al., "High-fiber rye bread and insulin secretion ad sensitivity in healthy postmenopausal women," *Amer Jour Clin Nutr* 2003; 77: 385–91.

Other books by

Pamela Wartian Smith, M.D., MPH

HRT—The Answers

A Concise Guide for Solving the Hormone Replacement Therapy Puzzle

Vitamins—Hype or Hope?

A Concise Guide for Determining Which Nutrients Work for You

Give the Gift of

DEMYSTIFYING WEIGHT LOSS

A Concise Guide for Solving the Weight Loss Puzzle

to Your Friends and Colleagues

CHECK YOUR LEADING BOOKSTORE OR ORDER HERE

❑ **YES**, I want _____ copies of *Demystifying Weight Loss* at $21.95 each, plus $4.95 shipping per book (Michigan residents please add $1.32 sales tax per book). Canadian orders must be accompanied by a postal money order in U.S. funds. Allow 15 days for delivery.

❑ **YES**, I am interested in having Dr. Pamela Smith speak or give a seminar to my company, association, school, or organization. Please send information.

My check or money order for $_________ is enclosed.

Please charge my: ❑ Visa ❑ MasterCard ❑ Discover ❑ American Express

Name ______________________________

Organization ______________________________

Address ______________________________

City/State/Zip ______________________________

Phone ______________ Email ______________

Card # ______________________________

Exp. Date __________ Signature ______________

Please make your check payable and return to:

Healthy Living Books, Inc.

907 Fisher Road • Grosse Pointe, MI 48230

Call your credit card order to: (313) 884-3229

Fax: (313) 884-3557

Order Online at: www.cfhll.com